TRANSFORMATIONS IN AMERICAN MEDICINE

Transformations in

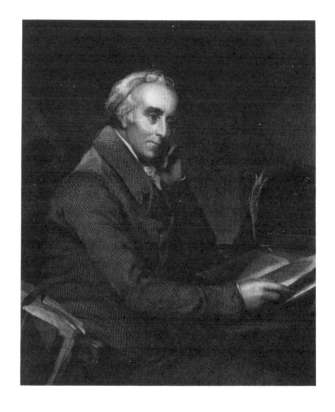

From Benjamin Rush

American Medicine

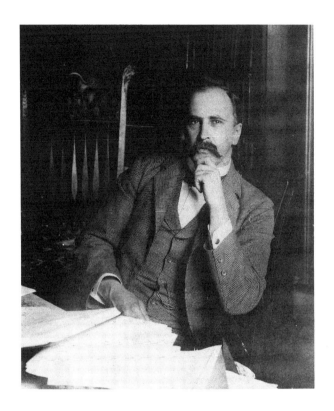

to William Osler

Lester S. King, M.D.

THE JOHNS HOPKINS UNIVERSITY PRESS
BALTIMORE AND LONDON

Publication of this book has been supported by a gift
from Chester Kerr made in honor of Steven Muller.

The Johns Hopkins University Press
701 West 40th Street, Baltimore, Maryland 21211
The Johns Hopkins Press Ltd., London

The paper used in this book meets the minimum requirements
of American National Standard for Information Sciences—Permanence
of Paper for Printed Library Materials, ANSI Z39.48-1984.

Library of Congress Cataloging-in-Publication Data will be
found on the last page of this book.

Title page illustrations: *left,* Benjamin Rush, from the Johns Hopkins Institute
of the History of Medicine; *right,* William Osler, from the Alan Mason Chesney
Medical Archives of the Johns Hopkins Medical Institutions.

Contents

TRANSFORMATIONS IN AMERICAN MEDICINE

1

A Survey of Relevant Problems

IN 1800, BENJAMIN RUSH (1745–1813) WAS THE OUT-standing physician in the United States. In 1900, William Osler (1849–1919), held a comparable position. A few similarities deserve notice. Both Rush and Osler, after receiving the best education available in their native lands, studied abroad and brought back the most advanced concepts and methods of their respective eras. Rush studied chiefly in Edinburgh, then the pinnacle of medicine, Osler in England and in central Europe, which was becoming dominant by the third quarter of the nineteenth century.

Both men immediately engaged in academic medicine and achieved great prominence as teachers. Rush taught in the newly founded University of Pennsylvania, the first medical school in the United States and for a century the outstanding school in the country. Osler taught first at McGill, in Montreal, and in 1884 became professor of medicine at the University of Pennsylvania, where Rush had preceded him. After four years there, he was selected to head the Department of Medicine at the new medical school at the Johns Hopkins University, soon to be the outstanding institution of its kind in the country. Through their own teaching and writing, and through their students, both men exerted a tremendous influence on medical education in their respective eras and, directly or indirectly, helped to train thousands of students and practitioners.

When each of them left active practice—Rush through death in 1813, Osler through voluntary retirement in 1905—medicine was in considerable turmoil. The era that, in a sense, culminated with Rush, was slowly crumbling as new attitudes and modes of thinking, new techniques and procedures, and new discoveries and concepts were gradually replacing the old. The once dominant structure, which we may call eighteenth-century medicine, was being replaced by a new edifice. Nineteenth-century medicine, like a medieval cathedral, took shape slowly over a long time span.

What I call nineteenth-century medicine, with Osler as its ideal representative, had no sooner reached imposing proportions than cracks began to appear in the fabric. New forces, slowly emerging, were gathering strength, to compel eventual radical change. In 1905, when Osler retired to Oxford, to become a much loved elder statesman, the profundity of the forthcoming changes was not yet apparent. But in retrospect we can see the massive transformation that occurred gradually in the twentieth century and rendered Oslerian medicine entirely obsolete.

TRANSFORMATIONS IN MEDICAL HISTORY

Medical theory follows a pattern of change, comparable to that in a living organism—tentative and uncertain entrance into existence; slow growth, often against difficulties and opposition; achievement of maturity and a period of dominance; and then decline, as new and competing theories enter the scene. There is a certain rough periodicity. Changes are gradual, perhaps imperceptible, over a short period, but they appear very striking when comparisons take place at longer intervals. Eighteenth-century medicine was transformed into the medicine of the nineteenth, but when seen in perspective, each had its own well-defined characteristics.

Any given moment sees a rise of the new and a decline of the old, although they take place at different rates. The well-known lines of O'Shaughnessy, written in 1881, are, I believe, applicable to medicine:

> For each age is a dream that is dying
> Or one that is coming to birth.[1]

In the present context, the sentiment refers to concepts, or modes of thinking, or values, or whatever measure we want for intellectual history.

This books deals with the way eighteenth-century medical concepts, as a coherent and once dominant body of doctrine, became transformed into what I call nineteenth-century medicine. By *century* I do not mean, literally, a hundred years. A medical era is characterized not by a particular number of revolutions around the sun but by trends, values, and events with no definite end point. A calendar provides only a rough framework for appreciating change.

I use the term *eighteenth century* to indicate a mode of thinking found predominantly (but not exclusively) within an arbitrary time span. The term correlates roughly with the attitudes embodied in the phrase Age of Reason or, in a different context, the Enlightenment. In literature, a comparable categorization might speak of the Age of Samuel Johnson. Historians of art or music might point to different groupings, and talk about the Age of Sir Joshua Reynolds or of Mozart.

By the later eighteenth century, upheavals were affecting virtually every branch of human endeavor, not only medicine but art, music, philosophy, law, literature, politics, and economics. As we pass from the era of Benjamin Rush to that of William Osler, we also pass from Haydn to Mendelssohn to Debussy, from Benjamin West to Delacroix to Monet, from cottage industry to factory production, from the oil or kerosene lamp to electricity, from the horse and wagon to the horseless carriage. Massive changes affected every cultural modality. The entire political, social, economic, and cultural fabric of the Western world was undergoing change. Epithets such as Romantic Movement or Industrial Revolution serve only as crude identifications and are not really very helpful.

In an earlier book, *The Medical World of the Eighteenth Century,* I presented my interpretation of eighteenth-century medicine, which extended from Herman Boerhaave (1668–1738) through William Cullen (1710–90) to Benjamin Rush and Samuel Hahnemann (1755–1843).[2] The succeeding era in medicine would comprise the environment in which William Osler grew up. This environment developed gradually and gathered strength as older trends declined. One rising curve overlapped another, declining curve. There was a crossing point, at which eighteenth-century thinking was largely but not entirely superseded by 19th-century thinking. This, I suggest, occurred in the 1840s. At that time, the older thought modes were still abundantly present but were already out of touch with the new progress.

Osler died in 1919. Within two decades of his death, the type of medicine that he represented was already out of date and the modes of thinking and of practice that had seemed so splendid at the turn of the century were rapidly becoming obsolete. And now, as we approach the twenty-first century, the same fate is overtaking the glories of the 1940s. New technology and new modes of thinking develop and foreshadow the obsolescence of a once proud dominion.

I am not propounding a theory of medical revolutions, for the existence of such events is indeed debatable.[3] Instead, I would emphasize the rhythm of change, which varies in intensity and velocity just as it does in biological growth and aging. Within this rhythm, I suggest, are broad patterns. The present book concentrates on one particular example of medical change, which began at the end of the eighteenth century, progressed through most of the nineteenth century, and entered senescence by 1900.

SOME NINETEENTH-CENTURY VIEWS

Throughout the nineteenth century, perceptive physicians realized that substantial changes were taking place. When we read their comments we learn more than merely the recorded data. We get a sense of values, of the things that medical leaders thought were important at that time; and we also gain insight into the personality of the writers and their relation to the times.

A splendid example of contemporary retrospection and evaluation we find in a lecture of 1851, published as a pamphlet with the title *Progress in Medicine During the First Half of the Nineteenth Century*.[4] The author, James Bryan, was professor of the institutes of medicine at the Philadelphia College of Medicine. His talk belonged to that interesting category known as Introductory Lectures, which a professor might give at the beginning of a course. He might not deal at all with the ostensible subject matter of the course but rather would discuss any topic that interested him. In this instance, Bryan, concerned with the history of medicine, reviewed for the students the medical progress of the preceding half century. He seemed quite aware that medicine was undergoing a change of direction, but the nature of that change was still obscure.

In describing new developments, his initial remarks have a thoroughly modern ring. He declared that "a physician educated twenty-five years ago, who has not by diligence and study kept up with the advances of science, could not now treat disease. . . . He would be obliged to study some of the elementary parts of his profession anew." This dictum educators have been repeating every generation, never more forcefully than today.

Bryan first discussed the influences carried over from the eighteenth century. The works of John Hunter and Xavier Bichat composed, he thought, a great scientific legacy, forming "the bases of all true medical reasoning." Another legacy was the spirit of independence, a tendency "to throw over all preexisting forms and set up those which were new." Gone into the discard, he said, were the nosology of Cullen and the theories of the "Solidists, Humoralists, and Chemists." The new century he regarded as "a young and ardent disciple of truth, who was welcomed to the New World and its wonders by the friendly hand of the venerable Rush." Worthy of notice here is the commendation of Rush, whom other commentators denigrated severely.

Then Bryan enumerated important medical figures of the first half of the century, taking up the progress by decades. In the first twenty years, the medical mind "was occupied in elaborating and perfecting the ideas of Hunter and Bichat" and applying them to the various aspects of medicine. He had in mind, apparently, the emphasis on observation and experiment. He noted the work of René-Théophile-Hyacinthe Laennec, "who [with his invention of the stethoscope] commenced and successfully prosecuted a new course of investigation and observations." So important had his contributions become that a physician who, in midcentury, "could not detect the normal and abnormal sounds . . . by means of auscultation and percussion, would be considered as at least thirty years behind the science of his day."

For the decade of the 1830s, Bryan mentioned the work of F. J. V. Broussias (1772–1838), whom we will take up in detail in a later chapter, and the rise of sects, such as the Thomsonians, the hydropaths, and the homeopaths. He also commented on the rise of microscopy, "after a long season of disuse," and the progress in anatomy and physiology.

Quite interesting were his views on the work of Justus von Liebig (1803–73), a leader in the new animal chemistry. We must appreciate the distinction between the old "Chemists," who had elaborated the iatrochemistry of the seventeenth and early eighteenth century and the newer experimental chemistry that was developing in the latter eighteenth century.[5] Liebig belonged to the new breed of scientists. He was applying the new concepts of chemistry, especially fermentation, to biological problems and infectious diseases.[6]

Liebig's work, Bryan thought, although "abounding in fanciful hypothesis," was being received "with acclamation" abroad. Combining existing knowledge with his own observations and experiments, Liebig had "woven a beautiful network of theory and fact." Bryan admitted the innovative approach "into hitherto unknown and unattempted regions." Yet, he added, whoever reads his works must carefully distinguish between conjecture and facts. Bryan seemed aware of the slowly progressing germ theory of disease, but he also apparently realized some of the attending logical pitfalls. (See chapters 7 and 8 for more on germ theory.)

Bryan's remarks on the decade of the 1840s were admittedly scanty, for he realized his own lack of desirable perspective. Of special interest is his comment that never before had there been such a profusion of books published on the various branches of medicine. He enumerated some of the writers he considered important. He noted, too, although briefly, the discovery of anaesthesia as one of the important events of the 1840s.

In reviewing Bryan's work, I note only those aspects that concern the present book. I deliberately omit his comments on surgery, therapeutics, and the various specialties.

Quite different were the historical comments of Elisha Bartlett (1804–55), whom we will meet repeatedly in these pages. Quite relevant here is an inaugural address given in 1841, when he became a professor at Transylvania University. He declared, "There has never been a time when we had as good cause for self-congratulation as we now have. . . . Never before . . . has it [medicine] made such rapid and sure progress as in the last forty years."[7]

Such a statement is surprising in view of the low esteem in which medical practice of the era is now regarded. Modern readers are led to believe that medical practice of the 1830s and 1840s, with its drastic bleedings and purgings, makes up a virtual horror story. We must distinguish, however, as does John Duffy, between the gradual accumulation of knowledge, and the "practice of the average physician," for whom the main question was not whether to bleed the patient, but only how much. The "disastrous results of heroic medical practice" contributed greatly to the rise of sectarian medicine.[8] John Warner, admitting the conventional view of heroic practice, provided a deeper analysis, as he carefully examined the gradual changes in therapy.[9]

Bartlett, in his retrospection, was concerned not with the every-day practice of medicine but rather with its "scientific" aspects. He had entitled his lecture "An Introductory Address on the Objects and Nature of Medical Science." He wanted students to know "the essential and true character of medical science . . . what are its objects of investigation, and what the true methods by which we can attain them."[10] These problems still engender lively dispute.

In the early nineteenth century, great progress was made in the philosophy of science, especially in France. Bryan virtually ignored this, while Bartlett called these conceptual advances to the attention of his students and colleagues. In 1844 he published a now classic text on the subject,[11] which I will discuss in chapter 8.

As a prime example of everything bad in medicine, Bartlett pointed to Benjamin Rush, of whose theories he declared, "It may be said, I think, that in the whole compass of medical literature, there cannot be found an equal number of pages, containing a greater amount of utter nonsense and unqualified absurdity."[12] His disdain was extended to William Cullen (1710–90), leader of the Edinburgh School, and John Brown (1755–88). Their doctrines, as we shall see, dominated medical theory and practice, as well as medical education, through the entire first third of the nineteenth century. Nevertheless, Bartlett expressly condemned them.

Pointing to the conceptual progress in medicine, he held up the French modes of investigation as the model of the future. (French medicine is explored further in chapters 5 and 8.) The older intellectual values were indeed being slowly replaced by new influences. Bartlett provided an evaluation and a critique, rather than a narrative exposition of progress such as Bryan had offered.

We get a rather different survey of the past from Austin Flint (1812–86), the leading American physician in the generation preceding William Osler. Flint was invited to present an address before the British Medical Association but died before the lecture could be delivered. It was, however, published as written.[13] The paper bore the intriguing title, "Medicine of the Future." Written in 1886, it first reviewed briefly the achievements of the preceding fifty years and then extrapolated the progress into the next fifty years, to predict what medicine would be like in 1936. (Interestingly enough, it was in 1888 that Edward Bellamy published his famous *Looking Backward, 2000–1888*. This utopian novel also extrapolated some of the scientific achievements but paid more attention to the social and political trends of his era. It is not possible to say at present whether the earlier work influenced the later.)

Flint dealt with three time periods. For the sake of symmetry, he went back fifty years to 1836, as a balance for the succeeding fifty years. However, he mentioned briefly the important discoveries of the nineteenth century prior to 1836. He considered as especially significant William Jenner's introduction of vaccination, Laennec's discovery of auscultation, Marie-François-Xavier Bichat's studies of general anatomy, and the work of Charles Bell and of François Magendie on the nervous system. Also falling within the period 1836–86 were other advances, including the knowledge of the nervous system and its functions, such as the localization of cerebral function; the numerical method (see chapter 8), which helped to produce statistical analysis; the great progress in microscopy; the discovery of anaesthesia; and thermometry. The place of honor, however, went to "the more recent revelations respecting the bacterial origin of disease."

Certainly, progress was vast. Flint quoted Sir James Paget, who, writing in 1881, said that in the preceding fifty years the progress of science was "twice as great as that in the previous fifty."[14] Judging by the past, said Flint, the advance in the next fifty years (to 1936) would be still greater.

Predictions for the future necessarily rest on the achievements of the immediate past. Furthermore, they indicate the type of activity that was most appealing at the time of writing and that seemed to have the greatest potential. In predicting the medicine of 1936, Flint paid special attention to chemistry. At the time he wrote, histology was "in the ascendent," a reference, perhaps, to the work of Rudolph Virchow. But in the next half century, he thought, organic chemistry would "penetrate dark recesses which histology cannot reach." The remarkable achievements with electricity, especially as related to the telephone, the phonograph, and the amplifier, greatly intrigued him. He thought it likely that in the future many abnormal conditions in the body could be studied by the sounds that they make.

In regard to pathology, he wrote that the "supreme objects of study" were the microorganisms and the way that they gave rise to the phenomena of disease. In the previous half century, great progress had been made in morbid anatomy, clinical descriptions and differential diagnosis, and the causal relations different affections had with each other. But the same progress could not as yet be said of etiology. Flint strongly hoped that the discovery of microorganisms would indicate the specific cause of infectious diseases.

Letting his imagination play, he pointed to the specific therapy in malaria. The disease was controlled "by remedies the efficacy of which is to be explained by their destructive effect on a specific organism"—and this even though "it is not certain that the parasite has yet been described." He thought it possible that all infectious diseases might be controlled as were the "malarial affections."

The paper is fascinating reading today, when Flint's target date has come and gone. It is not necessary to take up in detail additional points of emphasis that he described for his own time or projected into the future. With the wisdom of hindsight, we acquire from his work a background for evaluating the medical events of the latter nineteenth century and for understanding the transformations that would take place in the twentieth century.

MEDICAL THEORY AND MEDICAL PRACTICE

The three authors mentioned have, among them, given us a generous glimpse of the changes in medicine during the nineteenth century. We must, however, study a little more deeply the term *medicine*, which was used in different senses.

When someone becomes ill, there arise two distinct questions. First, *what* do you do for the patient? And second, *why* do you do it? Answers to the first question relate to therapy and compose the practice of medicine. Answers to the second question have an explanatory function and make up the theory of medicine. The practical and the theoretical aspects have different goals: in the one case, to heal the sick; in the other, to understand disease, explain its phenomena, expand our knowledge, and provide rationale for treatment. Obviously, practice and theory are closely related, but they have a certain fundamental independence.

This becomes apparent from linguistic derivation. The word *physician* comes from the Greek root *physis*, meaning nature. From the same root also come physiology, physics, and physicist. All the derivatives are intrinsically bound up with the phenomena of nature, whose study was originally part of philosophy. With specialization, there split off the branch called "natural philosophy," which then became "science." In the seventeenth century, natural philosophy was pretty much synonymous with what we now call physics but had no necessary connection with disease.

The phenomena of nature, as they concerned the human body, soon became *physiology.* To designate the phenomena of disease (in contrast to the normal) the word *physic* was used. Besides indicating a body of knowledge, the term extended its meaning to include the professional activity that dealt with such matters. The word *physician* meant a person who had studied physic, that is, the phenomena of disease, and who then might (but need not necessarily) engage in treating patients. The word *medicine* comes from the Latin *medere,* to heal. It now refers to either the substances used to promote healing or, by extension, the profession and art of healing.

The practitioner who engages in treating the sick may or may not understand the phenomena of disease—that is, be well grounded in physic. Even in antiquity there was a sharp difference between practitioners well educated in the science of their day and healers who practiced without that knowledge.

In the eighteenth century, two types of practitioners were clearly distinguished. Physicians, who had studied physic, had the knowledge to explain what they did and why they did it. On the other hand, apothecaries were practitioners who lacked that knowledge. While they engaged in the activity of healing, they did not have the "scientific" background that supplied the rationale for what they did. They had a lesser professional and social status and, in popular opinion, did not have the professional competence of the more learned physician.[15]

In the nineteenth century, this formal distinction was abolished.

All legally qualified practitioners were physicians. Apothecaries became general practitioners, physicians eventually became specialists.

Some physicians were especially concerned with the extension of knowledge and with clarifying areas hitherto obscure. Others were content to accept on faith the pronouncements made by the more learned. The new knowledge resulting from research had to filter down into the rank and file of practicing physicians. For the historian, this diffusion of knowledge provides special problems quite different from those relating to research as such and to the expansion of science. In this book, I will deal mainly with the latter.

As implied in the etymology of the terms *physic, physiology, and physician*, medical theory is particularly concerned with science. Medical practice at its best involves the application of science to individual patients. Medical practice at its worst ignores science and in treating patients relies sometimes on rules of thumb, sometimes on past experience without critical examination, sometimes on superstition and imagination. Any historical analysis of medicine must consider the nature of science and the different views that prevailed at different times. The subject forms a major component of this book, but for preliminary orientation I will indicate, in broad outline, the nature and scope of medical science as I interpret it.

The noted biologist Ernst Mayr offered an excellent definition. "Science," he said, "wants to explain, it wants to generalize, and it wants to determine the causes of things, events, and processes."[16] This succinct formulation is a fine operative definition. Although it does not mention medicine, it does tell us what medical science has tried to do: it concerns itself with general principles rather than particular cases, and it tries to explain observed phenomena through their causes.

This definition of Mayr's, centering on the generalized explanation of phenomena through their causes, will be the guiding thread as we explore the changes in American medicine. The various implications will receive detailed attention when we deal with concrete instances in the transformations. For the present, I will clarify a few of the general features and ideas that underlie the entire book.

THE CAUSAL RELATIONSHIP

The concept of cause plays a major role in any history of the science of medicine. Historically, the term has been used in different senses, or at least, with different implications. Since the cause of disease is so important in this book, I will offer here a preliminary orientation to some of the meanings of *cause* found in the medical literature of the past 200 or more years. (More detailed consideration is given in chapter 8.)

Aristotle, who identified four different types of causal relationship, provided the first systematic analysis. Later philosophers elaborated the subject with great subtlety, which for present-day students is perhaps more confusing than illuminating. By the early seventeenth century, however, leading physicians, still working in the Galenic tradition, had adopted a formulation that reflected the then prevailing state of knowledge.

They discriminated many different kinds of causal relation, each of which had a particular reference, generally self-explanatory: the cause per se and the cause per accidens; the principal cause and the adjuvant cause; the continuing cause; the proximal and the remote causes; the external and the internal causes; the cause sine qua non; the predisposing cause and the precipitating or exciting cause, and the like.[17] This proliferation gradually sorted itself out, and by the early nineteenth century the chief remaining categories were the remote and proximal causes and the predisposing and exciting causes. These concepts played an important role in eighteenth-century and nineteenth-century science and will be discussed in detail.

Today, at least in popular writing, the word *cause* is used quite uncritically, especially when combined with the word *exact*. We often read in the newspaper that investigators are searching for "the exact cause" of a particular fire—was there arson, or defective wiring, or carelessness with a cigarette? The answer, obviously, has important practical consequences, but only within a limited context. Older writers would have called this the search for the precipitating or occasional cause, recognizing full well that other types of cause were also operating. Modern writers tend to ignore this complexity, with its need for greater precision. Lacking this, confusion has resulted.

We cannot speak of *the* cause of an event, without qualification. The definite article *the* implies a singularity. We may correctly speak of *the* vice-president of the United States but not of *the* vice-president of General Motors. With multiplicity, the word *the* is totally inappropriate unless we use a qualifying term, such as the vice-president in charge of advertising.

So it is with cause. "The exact precipitating cause" makes sense, but "the exact cause," without further specification, does not. When we maintain that science explains phenomena through their causes, we must appreciate the multiplicity and interdependence of causal factors. Older physicians expressed this realization through the various qualifications they attached to the word *cause*. It will be our task to understand what these various qualifications meant in reference to disease.

Despite any difficulties, the knowledge of causes supposedly identified the good or "scientific" physician and distinguished him from the less competent. Chaucer, we recall, in describing the learned physician, included the statement, "He knew the cause of everich maladye." This special knowledge, discriminating the learned physician from the ordinary practitioner, provides a distinction that still applies today.

In this study of transformations in American medicine, I restrict myself largely to the theoretical and conceptual aspects. While this book covers the period from the heyday of Benjamin Rush to the retirement of William Osler, the range of topics is limited. The details of treatment or the practical aspects of medicine I deliberately avoid.[18] My concern lies with changing medical theory and what I call the conceptual foundations of medicine. And this aspect, in turn, relates closely to the notions of cause.

MODES OF THINKING

What we call medical advances, the actual concrete achievements, went hand in hand with changes in the ways of thinking— in attitudes toward evidence, in evaluations of relevance—all implicit in the ideas of causation. Most historical studies of nineteenth-century medicine attend to the achievements themselves. I want to examine, rather, modes of thinking that accompanied concrete advances.

The mind of Benjamin Rush seemed to work in channels quite

different from those that directed the thinking of William Osler. To characterize some of the differences, I repeatedly use the phrases "eighteenth-century thinking" and "nineteenth-century thinking." These terms cannot be defined now, for the whole book is devoted to expounding the meanings. The changes mentioned by Bryan, Bartlett, and Flint furnish, in a sense, the material through which conceptual changes were manifested.

The germ of this book insinuated itself into my mind some thirty odd years ago. In my first major study of the eighteenth century, I wrote a chapter on Samuel Hahnemann and his brainchild, homeopathy. "Hahnemann belonged, first and foremost, to the eighteenth century. He shared its limitations and prejudices, its attitudes and modes of thought. Although he had lived and worked for over forty years in the nineteenth century, he never progressed beyond his early environment."[19]

When Hahnemann died, his doctrines were already an anachronism in medical science, reflecting the thinking of a century before. Nevertheless, his ideas persisted through most of the nineteenth century and well into the twentieth, even though different standards were prevailing in medical circles. At that time, I did not pursue the differences, but now, some thirty years later, the then larval ideas have developed and find expression in this book.

SCOPE AND LIMITATIONS

To study the changes in medical thinking a sharp limitation of the field is obviously necessary. It is not feasible to study all diseases. I chose for detailed examination the group of febrile conditions called essential fevers. These, the major medical puzzle of the early nineteenth century, included what were called "continued" and "intermittent" fevers. Such a limitation gives a relatively homogeneous group, which logicians call a limited universe of discourse.

Moreover, I direct the analysis chiefly to the United States. This limitation allows us to study the entrance of European (including British) ideas and methods into new territory. We can then examine the growth and the changes such ideas underwent through the influence of the new environment. As the new country developed its own culture, medicine showed divergence from its origins in Europe.

Medical progress, originating in Europe, entered the United States through certain well-defined channels. One, physicians trained in Europe, especially in Great Britain, immigrated to the United States, bringing ideas and expertise with them. Two, Americans went to Europe to complete their education and brought back new expertise and new ideas that gradually diffused to the rest of the country. Three, medical books, especially those published in Great Britain, had a wide circulation in the United States, either through importation of the foreign editions or, more commonly, by republishing in this country. Texts chosen for reprinting had been written chiefly for a British audience. Sometimes American physicians would edit the works and add notes, or an appendix, or insertions in the text. The additions would usually relate to the differences that particular diseases might manifest in America and usually had to do with therapy. Translations of French and German texts were undertaken much less frequently.

Meanwhile, American authors were writing textbooks from their own experience. The 1840s witnessed a remarkable outpouring of books. Many medical works published at this time had a catalogue or publisher's list bound in at the end of the text. We can thus obtain a good idea of the quantity and scope of medical publications in midcentury.

Medicine offers a splendid opportunity to study the way ideas entered the United States and the way the environment affected medical practice and theory. During the period under consideration, the U.S. environment changed markedly and so, too, did all the components of medicine. We may fairly ask, how did these medical changes relate to the total environment?

In discussions of problems such as this, some historians have distinguished a viewpoint called internalism from another viewpoint called externalism, and characterize fellow historians as internalists or externalists. Internalists supposedly deal chiefly with conceptual matters. They "focus on the development of scientific ideas and theories, tracing their internal logic and conceptual linkages . . . and the degree of their evidentiary support." Externalists, on the other hand, "embed scientific ideas and theories in the human world. . . . They suppose that scientific ideas reflect only psychological complexes or social relationships."[20]

Restricting myself to medical history, I firmly reject this distinction, expressly and completely. Medicine forms a seamless unity with the total environment. There is an indissoluble interaction. I enthusiastically adopt the views of Rosen, who declared that "medicine is but one aspect of the general civilization of a period, expanded into a broad sociological context . . . within a matrix at once political, economic, social, and cultural."[21] I maintain that medical ideas—the principal concern of this book—have been influenced by social, cultural, economic, technological, and psychological factors (and any others that you may think of). They all interact, but we can study only one aspect, one particular set of relationships, at a given time.

Medical concepts I like to compare to living organisms. As they interact with the material environment, they undergo a process of building up and tearing down, a sort of metabolism. They grow, change, and then eventually decline. To prosper and spread, they require favorable conditions, which may be as complex as those affecting human nutrition. The various relevant factors that promote or hinder the growth of medical ideas may often be referred to well-recognized disciplines. Geography and demography have special relevance, clearly recognizable in the United States.[22]

The westward expansion provided medicine with an environment quite different from that obtaining in the cities of the East Coast. Urban and rural environments offer their own characteristics, and the so-called frontier provided a still different setting. In both practice and theory, the medical background of the metropolitan centers differed markedly from that of the frontier. Population density had a profound effect on the practice of medicine and on the normal growth (or metabolism) of medical ideas.

In sparsely settled areas, the provision of medical care offered various problems, important for any analysis of medical practice. For the study of medical theory, however, an especially significant feature is the character of medical education. Medical concepts are propagated through medical education, and this was markedly affected by demographic and economic factors.

A splendid example of these influences occurred in Ohio and Kentucky in the first few decades of the nineteenth century. These states (as representative of the whole district) underwent massive growth. Medical practice and medical education tried to keep pace. The story of Daniel Drake; the founding and decline of various medical schools, especially the rise and fall of Transylvania University; the diffusion of concepts, especially from Philadelphia; and the improvement in communication and the gradual urbanization all provide a magnificent example of the way that the environment helped to affect not only medical practice but also medical ideas over several decades.[23]

INTERACTIONS WITHIN MEDICAL HISTORY

American history furnishes a laboratory, so to speak, in which the intellectual history of medicine can readily be studied in relation to social, economic, geographic, demographic, and cultural components. Diffusion of influence, of course, was not merely a one-way passage. The cosmopolitan East was a locus from which ideas changed and spread westward, but the reverse current was not without effect, over a period of time.

As we study the growth and development of medical ideas, which compose what I consider the intellectual history of medicine, we constantly interact with what is commonly called the social history of medicine. Physicians enter into three kinds of interaction, each of which might be considered in isolation but which are essentially and indissolubly connected. First of all, we have the relationship between the physician and the patient, the realm of medical practice that has given rise to a subsidiary area generally known as medical ethics. In the present work, I will not enter into these fields.

Second, we have the relationship of the physician and nature. This is the realm of science whose goals are primarily understanding, explanation, and analysis of causes. The added advantage of such study is in the practical benefits it might yield.

Third, we have the interaction between physicians and the rest of society. The professional activities of physicians are intimately related to the pursuits of other individuals. These interactions involve economic, political, and ethical factors, which, in the broadest sense, compose the social history of medicine. Most of medical history written today would fall into this area. Medical institutions (medical schools and hospitals), the funding of medicine in its various activities, organizations of physicians into coherent social groups (associations, colleges, societies, academies, and the like), conflicts between medical groups and other social groups, and the growth of public policy in regard to medicine all are parts of social history.

The intellectual history of medicine, which emphasizes the conceptual basis, meshes with every other part of medical history. With this viewpoint, to call one aspect internal and another external is really meaningless. To be sure, the connections between medical ideas and other aspects of our culture may be more circuitous in some instances than in others, but the relationships exert an effect, nevertheless.

The ideal medical history would show, at all times, the relationship between the social and intellectual aspects of medicine. But the practical problems of exposition require sharp limitation. The present book aims to describe the actual changes in some medical ideas, in a limited time span, together with a few of the influences acting thereon.

CHANGES IN THE MEANING OF TERMS

One hindrance to the appreciation of the past lies with the changed meanings of terms. Many words used in the eighteenth and nineteenth centuries are still current in the medicine of today, but they do not mean the same now as they did then. As a few examples, I suggest *hypothesis, pathology, symptom, germ, fever, sympathy, typhoid, virus, and inflammation.* These were key terms in earlier medicine and still are today, but if in reading the older texts we interpret these words in the modern sense, we commit the cardinal sin in history—presentism. This means interpreting the past through the meanings and values of the present, instead of trying to understand the past in its own terms. Many writers who deride the thinking of a previous era are indulging in presentism. In this book, I pay attention to the meaning of the terms as used in their contemporary setting, and I try to describe the changes as they occurred over a century. In this way, we can reconstruct concepts as they gradually developed and, thereby, as they affected the entire medical context. In the next chapter I will discuss some of the basic terms of the eighteenth century, from which developed the concepts of the nineteenth century.

2

Some Basic Concepts
of Eighteenth-century
Medicine

THE MANTLE OF THE LEADING MEDICAL PROFESSOR
in the Western world descended from Herman Boerhaave to
William Cullen. The latter's major work, *First Lines of the Practice
of Medicine*, went through many editions.[1] In a preface dated November 1783, he provided a succinct account that can serve as a
watershed of change. He looked back to the earlier eighteenth
century and presented the medical concepts that had then prevailed. He also indicated his own evaluations and methodology,
helping us to appreciate the changes that would occur in the next
sixty years.

We can gain a good overview of eighteenth-century medical
concepts by emphasizing a few specific topics discussed in that
preface. These include the concepts of system and hypothesis, the
relations of reason and experience, and the nature of pathology.

PREOCCUPATION WITH SYSTEM

Even in the eighteenth century, the term *system* had several
distinct meanings, but all had the sense of order and of interconnec-
tion of parts that acted as a unit. This usage might refer to the body
as a whole, reacting as a physiological unit. Thus, quite commonly
we read that a drastic remedy achieved its therapeutic effect by
providing "a shock to the system." Such terminology made no
pretense to detailed knowledge but merely asserted a unified physiological activity, type undetermined.

Another important eighteenth-century usage had a conceptual reference, namely, the orderly arrangement of interrelated ideas and principles that described and explained phenomena. The scope might be enormously broad, as in the philosophical systems of Descartes, Leibniz, and Spinoza. Or, the ideas in question might have a more limited scope, as in medical systems, like those of Stahl, Hoffman, Boerhaave, and Cullen himself. These men organized the data of health and disease, showed inner connections and relationships, and provided explanations through a limited number of first principles.

In his preface, Cullen noted briefly the medical systems that had been influential in the first half of the eighteenth century. For substantive details, I refer to some of my earlier studies.[2] Here I will deal only with Cullen's critical observations that relate to the methodology of eighteenth-century medicine and the changes that would soon take place.

Conceptual systems such as those of Boerhaave and Cullen made first of all a laborious collection of "facts," which were organized to display orderly relationships. Then there were generalizations, whereby observations of "some" could be converted into statements about "all." And finally, the inferences must lead to broad first principles that would "explain" the individual data.

Some modern writers who heap ridicule on earlier conceptual systems as merely imaginative, ignore the empirical basis on which these systems rested. Actually, a system of medicine always starts with some sort of empirical observation and then, by logic, builds up a coherent body of generalizations and explanations. The system hangs together as a unit, so that changes in one part, even if apparently slight, might affect the whole. A physician who labored many years to construct a logical system in which everything fitted together would naturally be quite loath to change it.

Cullen fully credited Boerhaave's "excellent, systematic genius" and declared that his system was better than any that had preceded it. But Boerhaave, although he lived almost forty years after first forming his doctrine, "had hardly, in all that time, made any corrections of it, or additions to it," despite the extensive new information that had accumulated during that time.[3] Cullen pointed out several details wherein Boerhaave's statements had been shown incorrect by later observers.

However, if enough new facts came to light, these would require not a patching of the old system but the construction of a new one. New advances in medicine demonstrated the need for a new system. Cullen declared, "when many new facts have been acquired, it becomes requisite that these be incorporated into a system, whereby not only particular subjects may be improved, but the whole may be rendered more complete, consistent, and useful" (ibid., p. 17).

Cullen provided excellent arguments to show the necessity of systems. A leading French physician, Joseph Lieutaud (1703–80), had published extensive observations, but he had worked "on the plan of collecting facts, without any reasoning concerning their causes." The result Cullen regarded as disastrous, showing such a "total want of method, arrangement, system, or decision" as to be quite useless (p. 19). Masses of facts, alone, have no value: they must have organization, which requires the demonstration of interconnections and causal relationships, which in turn depend on reasoning and inference. Mere collection of facts, without any organization, was not enough. As Benjamin Rush later declared, facts, piled together, "would soon tumble to pieces, unless they were cemented by principles."[4]

The eighteenth-century systematists appreciated the importance of facts but also insisted that these be organized and brought into relation one with another. Only a system could achieve this desirable goal. Cullen wanted to create a system "that should comprehend the whole of the facts relating to the science," in a fashion better than had been done before.[5] He realized that his system would, like those that preceded it, require eventual change, but meanwhile he considered it the best available.

In the desire for a comprehensive system, the important term is not so much *system* as *comprehensive*. Cullen was on firm ground when he rejected the mere piling up of facts without the display of relationships. Today, medical students, facing infinitely more facts, crave an orderly arrangement that reveals the interdependence and causal relationships. A lecturer who provides such clarification is justly popular. He has, in eighteenth-century terms, reduced the data to a system.

Cullen, however, stood on shaky ground when (like his predecessors) he tried to embrace all of medicine in a single broad formulation. Of course, this "error" is apparent only in retrospect. In the seventeenth and eighteenth centuries, there was no good reason why a system should not be comprehensive. Various intellectual disciplines had long shown a tradition of such efforts, such as the *Summa* of St. Thomas. In secular philosophy, Descartes had introduced a new order when he propounded his own system, whose bases were thought and extension. But most important was the work of Sir Isaac Newton, who had created a single mathematical system that provided orderly explanation for terrestrial and celestial phenomena. He provided the ideal model and in so doing had won the approbation of all scientists and philosophers. Medical systematists tried to find a comparable formulation for the phenomena of health and disease.

This search for comprehensive explanations cast into a system did not cease with the end of the eighteenth century. In medicine in the early part of the nineteenth century, the most important example of system formation was homeopathy. In the twentieth century, orthodox Freudian psychoanalysis had all the characteristics of an eighteenth-century medical system.

CONDEMNATION OF HYPOTHESIS

Eighteenth-century thinkers distinguished two different kinds of foundation for a system. One stood firmly on observation and was elaborated through sound reasoning. The second type rested on the flimsy basis called hypothesis, a bad word indeed in the seventeenth and eighteenth centuries. Today, hypothesis is something praiseworthy, exuding special scientific virtue. The modern reader, therefore, may suffer a wrench in reversing his evaluation and in appreciating the older meaning of *hypothesis* as highly pejorative.

Isaac Newton expressed this viewpoint in his famous dictum, "Hypotheses non fingo." The key word here is *fingo*, root of our word fiction, that is, something created out of imagination. In the earlier usage, hypothesis was the equivalent of fiction, with only tenuous relation to facts. Newton was asserting firmly that his concepts were based on rigorous observation and, therefore, were not hypotheses. He denied that he was uttering fiction.

In the preface to *First Lines*, Cullen declared, with due pride, "I flatter myself that I have avoided hypotheses, and what have been called *theories*" (p. 23). In the eighteenth century, each systematist might criticize his predecessors for relying on hypotheses. He then might claim that he himself was not guilty of that fault but instead was employing sound and well-based reasoning. Cullen claimed that he tried to "establish many general doctrines, both physiological and pathological; but I trust that these are only generalization of facts, or conclusions from a candid and full induction."

REASON AND EXPERIENCE: METHODOLOGY

Eighteenth-century physicians were deeply concerned with facts that could be generalized through the exercise of sound reason. Error arose if the observations were inaccurate or perhaps insufficient, or if the reasoning was fallacious. Unfortunately, earlier physicians did not have any rigorous way of establishing a fact nor any effective criteria for evaluating the reasoning employed.

When later we take up in detail the analysis of fevers in the nineteenth century, we will gain a better idea of what observations the physicians accepted as fact and what forms of reasoning they considered valid (or *just*, to use the term popularized by Boerhaave). We will then see how the vagueness of eighteenth-century observations gradually acquired precision and the way critical judgment gradually expanded. In the older period, just as today, observation and reasoning are the bases on which all science rests. What has changed is the critical judgment that evaluates the observation and the reasoning.

Cullen started with observations and then derived general principles by what he thought was a "cautious induction." Reasoning, however, might be good or bad. Cullen believed that he himself engaged in proper reasoning. If, however, his inductions were not "cautious," then they would yield only hypothesis, or theory, and that was bad. What we call eighteenth-century rationalism thus had a twofold foundation: facts, the basis of all science; and reasoning, which transformed facts into general principles, or laws. With such a viewpoint, it would seem, no one should have any legitimate quarrel. But quarrel they did, and vehemently.

If we ask why eighteenth-century rationalism fell into disrepute, the answer relates in part to the changing meaning of terms. What is a fact, and how do you identify it? What is reason, and in what way does it function? Answers of the nineteenth century differed from those of the eighteenth. Similar transformation overtook the terms *cautious induction* and *sound reasoning.* Eighteenth-century rationalists committed the very faults they claimed they were avoiding. Their alleged facts were in large part not facts at all, their reasoning not cautious but wildly speculative. But at the time this was not apparent.

Leading theorists placed special importance on something called reason, however it might be defined. In contrast is another traditional term, *empiricism,* which implies a special dependence on something else, called experience. There is no real conflict between the two, for each requires the other. Experience provides observation, the facts, the content on which reason works. Reason brings order into experience through inference, generalization, concepts, and in a more elaborate fashion, theories. Kant phrased the relationships by saying that precepts without concepts were blind, concepts without precepts were empty. Each is unthinkable without the other, in the same way that the word *inside* is meaningless without the word *outside.* The words *empiricism* and *rationalism,* however, have acquired subsidiary meanings. The cognate terms *empiric, empiricist,* and *empirical* have variable connotations, which I will identify later. For the present context, I use *empiricism* as it applies to Hippocrates, Sydenham, Bacon, and Locke, who were specially concerned with observation and modest low-level inferences. Other meanings will appear later.

Eighteenth-century systematists, who all paid homage to observation and facts, might be called empiricists. Since they also lauded the power of reason to achieve truth, they could also be called rationalists. The distinction between the two rested on degree and emphasis. How much observation did you need for the inferences you made? Did you have enough facts to support your inferences? If inferences outran facts, you would end with hypothesis, and then the rationalism was excessive and bad. On the other hand, if too much attention was paid to facts, as Cullen accused Lieutaud of doing, then empiricism was excessive and bad.

One great difference between eighteenth- and nineteenth-century thought lies in an altered view of how much was enough. Statements and inferences that seemed entirely adequate and acceptable at one time were later rejected as without foundation. Criteria of validity changed. What I call nineteenth-century thought modes relied on standards of validity quite different from those of the eighteenth century.

New criteria are accepted only slowly. For example, eighteenth-century systematists praised Francis Bacon no less than did the later empiricists, who derided the systematists. And although Bacon enunciated his doctrines in the early seventeenth century, and later in that century became the patron saint of the Royal Society, his ideas did not really take hold until well into the nineteenth century.

The great physicians of the era, like Boerhaave and Cullen, would not have classified themselves as rationalists. A strict disjunction between rationalism and empiricism gives an entirely false picture of the era. The real disjunction lay in the attitudes and way of thinking. The same words recur in different periods but have changed their meaning. Eighteenth-century writers condemned reasoning that went beyond the evidence, just as we do today, but the standards were different.

Older authors explicitly described what they meant by reason. Early in the eighteenth century, Herman Boerhaave gave an operative definition of *reason*. It was through reason, he said, that "the data of experience are tested, examined in all their characteristics, then scrupulously compared with each other, to reveal the agreements and differences; and then, most cautiously, everything is noted that is clearly implicit therein and can be inferred therefrom."[6]

Boerhaave was pointing to two distinct but related activities. The first was the examination of the data in order to determine similarities and differences, which were then compared and evaluated. Plato would have called this, distinguishing between the Same and the Other, an activity that requires comparison and discrimination. All this I would call the *critical function* of reason.

However, when data are already at hand, reason can go beyond the immediately given and try to find what the data imply. This it does through the process of inference, which elicits new truth from available information. Through inference, reason can point to causes, achieve generalizations, make abstractions, create theories, and reach first principles. It was this function that eventually would build systems. For this aspect I suggest the descriptive term, *constructivist function* of reason.

We find a comparable distinction half a century later, in the work of Thomas Percival (1740–1804), famous for his later treatise on medical ethics. In 1765 he wrote two essays, one arguing "against the use of theory and reasoning in physic"; and the other arguing for their use.[7] The mode of presentation was, in a sense, a rhetorical device for driving home an important distinction.

In the first essay, Percival pointed to the excesses of reason. He condemned rationalists because they indulged in empty theories and depended on imagination rather than fact. In contrast, he praised empiricism in medicine and indicated its proper function, namely, "to watch with close attention the operations of nature, to treasure up a store of useful facts, to learn by accurate observation the diagnostics of diseases, and by unbiased experience, the true method of cure." Ostensibly, he was condemning rationalism. But this was only part of the story.

In his following essay, Percival changed his approach and showed how the collection of facts by itself could lead to severe error, which could be corrected only through reason. In this context, reason was thus essential to medicine. The rationalist deserved praise, because he "attends diligently to nature in her operations, he selects and arranges facts and deduces general conclusions, and thus forms a consistent, rational, and useful theory on which his practice is built." Understanding of disease demands theory, which reason alone can provide. In this sense, *theory* is not at all a pejorative term but rather an essential component of science.

The writings of Cullen reflected both of these viewpoints. Although he did not provide any specific analysis, he made every effort to give us a well-balanced presentation of both experience and reason, and he was often explicitly critical when he discussed theoretical features of medicine. He stressed the need for observation and maintained that sound data would, through sound reasoning, lead to general principles. These, besides having explanatory value, could also serve to regulate practice. Yet by modern standards he was often "jumping to conclusions" on the basis of insufficient data. Moreover, as we now know, the data that he accepted were in large part severely flawed. The historian, of course, cannot fault him for not knowing what was not known. Much more important in intellectual history is Cullen's judicious attitude and his absence of dogmatism.

PATHOLOGY: CONCERN WITH DISCRIMINATION AND ETIOLOGY

The functions of reason had their greatest application in pathology. Today, this term is irretrievably bound up with autopsies, microscopic diagnosis, and laboratory examinations. The pathologist who understands these things provides the clinician with specialized information not otherwise available. Unfortunately, the modern reader who has absorbed this viewpoint may be baffled by the usage of *pathology* in the earlier literature.

For a useful baseline, I will use the definition that Boerhaave provided.[8] Pathology, he declared, treats "of Diseases, their Differences, Causes, and Effects, or Symptoms, by which the human Body is known to vary from the healthy State." This is so succinct, and so crammed with important concepts, that it needs considerable expansion.

Diseases are multiple. Pathology, in Boerhaave's view, had the initial task of making some kind of separation between them. At first the discrimination would be only approximate, but with increased knowledge large categories would become subdivided into smaller and more precise groups. The physician would search for defining features that could identify an individual condition and distinguish it from others that might be more or less similar.

The original criteria through which diseases were distinguished came first from bedside observation. The physical appearance of the patient provided important information and so did changes in function. A patient who was hot and flushed, had difficulty in breathing, a cough, and pain in the chest, presumably had a quite different disease than did a patient who was paralyzed on one side or a patient who had great difficulty in swallowing and had become emaciated.

The practitioner, to treat a patient intelligently, had to have some notions regarding the kind of disease involved. This required discrimination, which in turn depended on observation, reflection, and evaluation. These processes were part of pathology, the essence of medical science. Science came into being because physicians had observed, reflected, discriminated, and evaluated the available data and then come to a reasoned conclusion. All this is involved when we speak of pathology as the science of medicine.

This process of discrimination led eventually to the formal classification known as nosology, a term that historically falls into the realm of pathology, and which we will take up in detail later. Unfortunately, through misplaced exuberance and the poor critical judgment of some pathologists, nosology became an object of derision. Nevertheless, the functions it serves have retained their essential importance and are as significant today as in the eighteenth century.

Boerhaave recognized that medical science—pathology—included the discriminatory process, with the separation and identification of diseases. This was carried out by physicians who, in addition to treating the patient, tried to analyze the nature, causes, and relations of disease. In their activity as pathologists, who discriminated among diseases, they would use whatever data became available. Eventually, this would involve morbid anatomy, chemistry, physiology, bacteriology, epidemiology, and a host of other disciplines. All this fitted into the eighteenth-century concept of pathology.

The determination of causes is perhaps the most essential feature of pathology, and the task has engaged the attention of physicians since antiquity. The present-day association of pathology with autopsy examination has, unfortunately, obscured this true historical sense.

In seeking the causes of disease, medical scientists use whatever concepts are prevalent in their particular era. This is true today and was equally true in the eighteenth century. Originally, the data on which the pathologist depended came from bedside observation of the patient, together with the history that the patient might supply. As far back as Hippocrates, the physician also noted environmental factors that might have relevance in the production of disease. Galen codified many such factors, which became known as the nonnaturals.[9] In the eighteenth century, these played a considerable part in explaining the etiology of disease, but by the nineteenth century they had been absorbed into other categories and will not receive special discussion here.

Pathology, relying on the known causes of disease, also tried to explain the sequential steps by which any given disease became manifest. Today, this process is known as pathogenesis, whose explication has always been the function of the pathologist. In modern terminology, the etiology of disease identifies the various causal factors that are operative, while pathogenesis explains the ways in which these factors interact to produce the disease. The analysis of febrile diseases, discussed in the next several chapters, illustrates the relationships of these terms.

Since the etiology and pathogenesis of disease is the traditional domain of pathology, we may properly ask, what is the role of the postmortem examination? Where and how does the subject of morbid anatomy enter into the science of pathology? Cullen clearly indicated the eighteenth-century viewpoint. He declared that "in establishing a proper Pathology, there is nothing that has been of more service than the Dissection of morbid bodies." And this, he went on, "is chiefly valuable upon account of its leading us to discover the proximate causes of diseases."[10]

Although Cullen himself had little personal experience with dissection, he realized that this could furnish valuable information on the causes of disease. However, morbid anatomy was only one source of relevant data that might contribute to the knowledge of causes. It provided useful information to facilitate the study of causes, but the findings had to be critically evaluated. This need sharpened the skills of the pathologist. In the last third of the eighteenth century and the first two-thirds of the nineteenth, the influence of morbid anatomy expanded markedly and greatly affected the meaning of pathology.[11]

SIGNS AND SYMPTOMS

A third component of pathology, in the eighteenth-century sense, had to do with the signs and symptoms of disease. According to Boerhaave, the pathologist must study not only the causes of disease but also the effects. He used the word *symptom* as synonymous with *effect,* a usage continuing the tradition that went at least as far back as Galen, namely, that a symptom was any manifestation of disease. Only in the late nineteenth century did the stultifying confusion arise that a symptom was something that the patient was also aware of and a sign was something that only the physician could detect. When we study the various transformations in the nineteenth century, we will see how this confusion arose. In present-day medicine, the usage is so widely accepted that it would be quixotic to attempt its correction. Nevertheless, the original meanings must be clarified to keep the older writings from appearing nonsensical. For the historian, it is the present-day usage that is nonsensical.

In eighteenth-century medical science, there was a major subject called semeiology that dealt with signs. A sign points to something. It provides meaning and significance. It leads from the immediately given to something else. In medicine, a symptom becomes a sign if it points to some disease or disease state.

The distinction between symptom and sign relates to point of view. Pathologists, concerned with the conceptual aspects of disease, analyze its manifestations to understand its nature and the way it expresses itself. These manifestations are the symptoms, and a distinction into subjective and objective is pointless. Practitioners, on the other hand, called on to treat patients, must first determine (at least, approximately) the particular disease they are going to treat. Therefore, they study the symptoms to find out where they point, and when they point in a particular direction, they become signs. Practitioners must interpret these findings (i.e., convert symptoms into signs) and thus determine what disease they might indicate.

This conversion of symptoms into signs can be a science, which older physicians recognized and called semeiology. It dealt with the significance the symptoms might have and what diseases they might indicate, or at least suggest. During the nineteenth century, this venerable aspect of medical science underwent a change in name, to physical diagnosis. At first this was closely allied to pathology, and for a time some pathology texts included sections on the interpretations of signs.

THE IMPORTANCE OF MORBID ANATOMY

During the nineteenth century, the increasing number of autopsy examinations played an important part in eventually changing the concept of pathology. This took place partly through the process of diagnosis.

Diagnosis—the identification of a disease—depended on the observation and interpretation of symptoms, that is, manifestations of disease. The clinician could directly observe changes on the surface of the body, but manifestations occurring inside the body, hidden from sight, had to be inferred. Any such inferences depended largely on functional changes induced by the disease. Altered function was a manifestation of disease. Thus, difficulty in breathing would ordinarily be correlated with disturbances of the lungs or the heart; difficulty in urination, with the bladder or kidneys; paralysis or stupor, with the nervous system; and so on.

Early physicians, in contrast to surgeons, dealt especially with conditions affecting the internal organs (the designation *internal medicine* is still current today, although its origin is rarely considered). In clinical examination, what was happening in the interior of the body remained a matter of inference. A dissection, however, would open the internal organs to direct observation. Postmortem dissections greatly expanded the total amount of information that might have some relevance to the diagnostic process.

Study of early autopsy records is quite illuminating. In 1679, Theophile Bonetus (1620–89), in his *Sepulchretum*, compiled almost 3,000 autopsies recorded up to that time (see ibid.). This volume reveals to us what at that time was considered important in anatomical observation, the degree to which the anatomical findings helped (or failed to help) explain disease, and incidentally, what physicians thought about the nature of disease.

When we read the old reports, we find that most features that interest us today were simply not recorded. To some degree, this might have been due to lack of skill in observing and describing. But in all likelihood, most of what was seen was simply not considered worthy of note. There was no perception of relevance, no sense of connection between discrete phenomena. The sense of pattern was poorly developed.

Cullen, although he performed few if any autopsies, was a pathologist according to the then current usage. He studied the phenomena of health and disease, analyzed their causes, and elaborated a system of concepts that explained the phenomena. These concepts rested on certain first principles, not given directly in experience but inferred therefrom. In his explanations, he paid special attention to the concept of causes. This represented the essence of pathology. Morbid anatomy, although recognized as a worthwhile discipline, had a subordinate and accessory role.

We can see how completely this meaning disappeared when we examine the generally admirable and now classic work of Esmond Long, *A History of Pathology*.[12] Long did not even mention Cullen as a pathologist. The older explanatory concepts, so central in the tradition of pathology, Long dismissed as "speculative," a term of condemnation. It implied an absence of adequate "facts" and a reliance on imagination. By modern standards, earlier explanatory principles (such as the "spissitude" or "alkaline acrimony" of Boerhaave) may indeed appear totally imaginative. The historian, however, appreciates the empirical basis of the older theories.

Writers of the eighteenth and early nineteenth centuries must not be judged by modern usage. The older period had its own views on what constituted speculation, to which the eighteenth-century term *hypothesis* was applied. Just as Long condemned seventeenth- and eighteenth-century writers as speculative, so too did Cullen (among others) condemn many earlier writers for the same fault. Meanwhile, Cullen explicitly denied being tainted in this fashion.

G. B. MORGAGNI AND MODERN PATHOLOGY

Giovanni Battista Morgagni (1682–1771) is commonly called the first great pathologist. Historically, however, he should be regarded rather as the first great morbid anatomist. The two terms are not at all synonymous.

Morgagni was a many-sided physician, outstanding in several different areas. He was a leading clinician, that is, practitioner of medicine. Furthermore, he was an eminent anatomist, in the finest Italian tradition. Moreover, he was a pathologist, in that he wanted to explain diseases through knowledge of their causes and mechanisms. He was not, however, concerned with creating a comprehensive system or with elucidating first principles.

These latter features we commonly associate with the rationalism of Georg Ernest Stahl, Friederick Hoffmann, Boerhaave, and to a somewhat lesser degree, Cullen. Morgagni, on the other hand, played an important part in the new empirical trend, which conflicted with the older rationalism, gradually replaced it, and eventually dominated the medicine of the nineteenth century.

As a leading anatomist of his day, Morgagni's great technical skill in dissection and his capacity for precise observation and description led him to original discoveries in normal gross anatomy. His skill in dissection and his unrivalled knowledge of normal structure also made him preeminently fitted to study morbid anatomy. Furthermore—this is an independent feature—when he sought to clarify the nature of disease, he also showed excellent judgment and a capacity for sound inference.

His great book, *The Seats and Causes of Disease, Investigated by Anatomy,* is one of the masterpieces of medical literature.[13] The title itself tells much of what he was trying to do as well as the concepts and methodology of the times.

Since disease was understood principally in terms of disturbed function, the disturbance should be particularly manifest in some primary location. The disease process, once initiated, could spread to other parts of the body through the phenomenon of sympathy. Morgagni arranged his presentation by regions of the body, such as head, thorax, abdomen, and extremities. Each region harbored many organs, and each organ could be the seat of various diseases. Involved here is a presupposition that impaired function would go hand in hand with some sort of structural abnormalities in the affected organs. Such morbid changes would, by inference, indicate the site of the disease and perhaps its nature.

Anatomical study could also throw light on the causes of diseases as well as their site. Physicians accepted several different kinds of cause, such as proximal and remote, predisposing and precipitating, among others. The whole complicated subject will receive detailed analysis later. Suffice it here to emphasize the limitations that Morgagni made explicit, namely, the causes of disease studied by anatomical investigation. Only certain kinds of cause could be observed by this method. A miasma, for example, could be an exciting cause of certain diseases, and a particular diathesis or idiosyncrasy might be a predisposing cause, but neither of these could be investigated by anatomy in the sense that Morgagni used. Their investigation would require other methods.

In Morgagni's work, the causes revealed in dissection reflected direct observation. They differed from other, alleged, factors, like acrids or corrosive particles, which had earlier been asserted but had not been directly observed. The great merit of his book is the precise detail in which he described what he actually saw. The exact relationship that these changes would bear to the origins of disease would be hammered out in the future.

Morgagni's usage of the word *cause* raises some knotty points in the philosophy of science. For example, What is the disease of which this or that factor is alleged to be a cause? What constituted a disease entity? These problems are, I believe, implicit in Morgagni's work, but their significance will emerge only when we take up, in a later chapter, some specific febrile diseases.

Morgagni's exposition exhibits some special merits. He showed an encyclopedic knowledge of the relevant literature (and we today should realize what an enormous mass of descriptive literature was available in the eighteenth century). Then, as befits a good clinician, he usually gave a detailed clinical history. Furthermore, his description of anatomical changes at the "seat" of the disease was masterly and has aroused admiration from generations of pathologists.

A further component, quite significant in the present context, has received little attention heretofore. When the data were especially complex, Morgagni subjected the facts and assertions to critical evaluation. The descriptions found in the literature did not necessarily agree with his own, and a given disease condition might have a broad range of structural changes. Different examples of a disease, clinically the same, might show a considerable variety of findings. The relationship of morbid anatomy to the clinical phenomena might be obscure. Morgagni weighed the evidence and, from a critical evaluation, would reach his conclusions. These, he admitted, were probable only, and he avoided dogmatism. As a typical example, I would cite his discussion of palpitation of the heart and its relationships to affections of the pericardium.[14]

Morgagni devoted much effort to answering the questions, Where is the disease?, and What causes it? But the question, What *is* the disease?, he tended to avoid. Consistent with this attitude, he also avoided nosology and questions regarding the specificity and classification of disease. When he talked about individual ailments, such as gout, or phthisis, or apoplexy, or lues, he was falling back on popular and commonly accepted usage. He did not try to define individual diseases or relate them to each other. However, by pointing to precise anatomical correlates, he contributed to the understanding of disease and, hence, to their ultimate better definition and relationships.

In his work, Morgagni provided only very limited generalizations. On a case-by-case basis, he described what he saw, correlated his findings with the clinical picture, and provided a fine critical evaluation of evidence. His inferences always remained quite close to the concrete data. He did not make broad inductive leaps.

Knowledge of morbid anatomy and its correlation with function became increasingly important. Diagnosis of disease relied on symptoms, which generally called attention to disturbed function. Clinicians would locate diseases in one or another part of the body. On clinical grounds, the patient might have a disease of the brain, or the heart, or the stomach, but precision would be difficult. Any abnormal structure changes, disclosed at autopsy, that could correlate with the clinical impression would help to identify the site of the disease. Morgagni was a master in correlating clinical findings with the anatomical changes he observed in dissection.

Only a skilled clinician could appreciate the relationships that we now call the clinico-pathological correlation. As an outstanding anatomist, Morgagni provided vastly more accurate and complete descriptions than had his predecessors. And because he was an excellent clinician, skilled in interpreting symptoms, he could correlate the anatomical findings with the clinical findings better than any of his predecessors.

The intellectual history of medicine must consider the questions, What did the earlier physicians regard as important? What did they accept as fact? What connection did they believe one fact might have with another? Morgagni brilliantly reflects the changing background of the late eighteenth century. He was part of the cutting edge that was carving a new empirical approach to medicine. He was a key figure in the transition from eighteenth-century thinking to that of the nineteenth century.

3

*Inflammation
and Fever*

A T THE END OF THE EIGHTEENTH CENTURY, FEVER and inflammation were the most important "diseases" that the physician had to face. Today we regard these conditions not as discrete diseases but rather as reactions or symptoms, as components of a larger picture. To understand the earlier views we must resolutely put aside our modern ideas and enter into the frames of reference then prevailing. Physicians had to explain observed phenomena, without any knowledge of cell theory or bacteria, and with only the most rudimentary microscopy. Fever and inflammation were deemed separate yet in some way related. When we study the earlier theories and explanations, we must appreciate the level of knowledge then prevailing.

The manifest phenomena of both fever and inflammation had been well recognized since antiquity. William Cullen provided a succinct analysis. When, he said, the surface of the body "is affected with unusual redness, heat, pain, and tumor, we have the disease inflammation." Celsus, in the first century A.D., first described these so-called cardinal signs—tumor, rubor, calor, dolor—which present-day medical students still memorize. According to Cullen, when these findings are "considerable," they are accompanied by fever.[1]

Inflammation on the surface, directly and readily observed, was diagnosed by inspection. But when the internal organs were involved, direct inspection was not possible, and in such cases diagnosis was far more difficult. Of the classical diagnostic criteria, only pain could then be recognized with assurance. However, in internal inflammation, a further feature might be quite important, namely, a disturbance of function. Cullen would diagnose inflammation of the internal organs if there were "a fixed pain in any internal part, attended with some interruption in the exercise of its function" (ibid., par. 236). Today, in addition to the four cardinal signs of inflammation, some medical students add a fifth criterion, *functio laesa,* impaired function.

What we today would call laboratory examination also played a part in the diagnosis of hidden inflammation. In certain types of inflammatory disease, the blood, when drawn by venesection, shows phenomena to which earlier physicians paid special attention. A firm clot might form rapidly, with strong retraction and quick expression of the serum. There could also be a "buffy coat," corresponding to an increased number of white blood cells entrapped in fibrin. These phenomena we today associate with an increased sedimentation rate and leucocytosis. In an older period, study of the blood removed at phlebotomy could aid diagnosis, comparable to the way we now gain diagnostic information from a white blood cell count and the sedimentation rate.

PROXIMAL CAUSE

Just as we do today, earlier physicians tried to identify the essential nature of inflammation and fever and the "causes" that induced them. With an insight that puts many modern physicians to shame, earlier writers fully appreciated the complexity of the causal relationship. They avoided the error of referring to *the* cause of a phenomenon. Instead, they emphasized the multiplicity of factors and identified different components by individual names. In this chapter I will take up only a part of the analysis and will discuss other aspects in their appropriate contexts. Here I will touch on two factors, the proximal (or proximate) cause and the remote causes. These terms, although outmoded today, hold the utmost importance in any historical analysis.

The proximal cause indicated the functional aspects or physiological equivalents that underlay the disease or its symptoms. For any biological phenomenon, the proximal cause described the essential nature and the physiological activities that compose it. In inflammation, the proximal cause would be those bodily mechanisms that produced the cardinal signs already noted. Remote causes, on the other hand, would be the factors that led to the proximal cause.

To clarify proximal cause in present-day terms, I suggest as illustration the well-known experiments of Walter B. Cannon, carried out in a totally different context. He identified the physiological responses in cats when states of rage or fear were experimentally induced. He described the reactions in the autonomic nervous system and the endocrines, especially the adrenal medulla, when cats, in restraint, were exposed to barking dogs.[2] In an earlier nomenclature, these physiological changes would be, roughly, the proximal cause of the observed behavior; conversely, the observed behavior would be manifestations of these physiological changes. The behavior of the frightened cat and the underlying physiological correlates accompany each other like the two sides of a coin. Cannon demonstrated what was going on inside the body in particular patterns of behavior. He indicated in precise physiological terms the proximal cause of rage and fear.

Many different factors might bring this proximal cause into action and thus induce the observed behavior. All such inciting factors would be remote causes of the phenomenon in question. In Cannon's experiments, the exposure of the cat to a barking dog, under controlled conditions, was the actual remote cause, but there might be innumerable other situations.

If we return now to disease and ask the question, What *is* inflammation?, we are trying to find out what is going on inside the body when this observed phenomenon is present. We are seeking the proximal cause. Different pathologists gave different answers, but they all purported to describe the physiological processes found in inflammation. These changes would be the equivalent of the clinical disease but were expressed in other terms.

Inflammation, clinically observed, indicated a local accumulation of blood. More blood was flowing into a part than was flowing out. Boerhaave, writing in the heyday of mechanical philosophy, believed in some kind of physical impedance or the mechanical blockage, whether from increased viscosity of the blood or actual aggregates of corpuscles acting as plugs. According to this view, inflammation resulted from changes in the contents of the blood vessels.

Cullen rejected this mechanical interpretation and explained the phenomena of inflammation by reference to the solids rather than the humors. He stressed the active role of the blood vessels themselves, rather than their contents, and emphasized the importance of the nervous system. In any bodily part, an inflammation, he said, resulted from "an increased impetus of the blood in the vessels of the part affected." And this, in turn, was due to "the increased action of the vessels of the part itself."[3] To understand what this means, modern readers must place themselves in an eighteenth-century frame of reference.

The heart, acting as a pump, drove the blood through the vascular system, aided by the "action" of the vessels. By feeling the pulse, the physician could easily recognize changes in the action of the heart. It could be feeble or tumultuous, fast or slow, with corresponding changes in the impetus of the blood.

The arteries play an important part in the circulation of the blood. Cullen noted local variations. At different times "the velocity and impetus" of the blood "was unequal" in different parts of the body, "while the action of the heart continues the same."[4] Since the action of the heart was uniform, local variations would necessarily be due to changes in local blood vessels. If the heart showed no evidence of increased activity, local inflammation could be traced to changes in the local vessels themselves.[5]

But what were these changes? In Cullen's explanations, the key terms were "action of the vessels" and "spasm" of the "extreme vessels." The term *action*, in this context, referred to a contraction. The larger arteries were known to contain muscle fibers, and contraction of the large vessels could be directly observed. For the smaller vessels, however, there was no direct knowledge regarding their structure or functional activity. Lacking direct evidence, physicians resorted to extrapolation: the observed properties of the large vessels were simply assumed to extend to the finer and finer vessels.

According to Cullen's views, in every inflammation there is an "increased action of the vessels" of that part (ibid., par. 241). Increased action meant some degree of contraction. Narrowing of the lumen, it was well known, increased the velocity of flow, or impetus; impetus of blood seems to have been synonymous with quantity of blood.

When an "unusual quantity of blood" enters a part, through the increased impetus, "the extremities of the arteries do not readily transmit the unusual quantity of blood impelled into them." While this would be a general principle of hydrodynamics, in inflammation there was a "preternatural resistance to the free passage of the fluids" (par. 242). This abnormal resistance results from a spasm of the extreme vessels.

How and why an increased action, leading to an increased impetus, should under certain circumstances induce a spasm was not entirely clear (par. 243). We can say only that, in Cullen's views of inflammation (as was also true of fever), spasm provided an essential protective mechanism, operating through the *vis medicatrix naturae,* or healing power of nature.

A locally heightened action of the vessels might temporarily increase the local quantity of blood as a transitory phenomenon. To constitute an inflammation, this increased action must be maintained. This would be accomplished by an increased action of the more distal vessels, resulting from spasm at their extremities. This distal constriction, by increasing the resistance to flow, would intensify the "action" of the more proximal vessels. Said Cullen, "A spasm in the extreme arteries, supporting an increased action in the course of them, may therefore be considered as the proximal cause of inflammation" (par. 245).

REMOTE CAUSES

For a sound explanation, the pathologist must then show what induced an increased action of vessels in the first place. Here we enter the realm of remote causes. Cullen listed them under several heads (pars. 262, 253). He noted various "stimulant" agents. These included fire and burning heat; external violence, which produced wounds and mechanical damage; and also substances that, through their chemical "acrimony" or mechanical configuration, would act as an "irritant." All these would account for inflammations observed on the surface of the body.

Two other categories seemed especially concerned with internal inflammation. One major remote cause was "cold." This, according to current doctrine, would induce various kinds of internal inflammation, such as rheumatism, nephritis, bronchitis, or encephalitis. These represented diseases of an inflammatory nature. In one or another form, the notion that cold has a causal role in many internal diseases has persisted to the present day.

In some ways Cullen cloaked his ignorance by tautology. He gave as one cause "an increased impetus of the blood" in some particular area. This merely restates the original definition. If inflammation *is* an increased impetus of the blood, then whatever induces that increase will "cause" an inflammation. Eventually, these unknown factors would become concretely observable, for example, with the demonstration of bacteria.

Cullen's emphasis on "action" and "spasm," however vague, had an important implication. It meant the rejection of simple mechanical explanations and the acceptance of a "vital" activity related, somehow, to the physiology of the nervous system. Today, vitalism is regarded as a retreat into obscurantism, but when Cullen wrote, and for a long time thereafter, this was not so. A recourse to vitalism showed that the explanations based on prevalent theories of physics and chemistry no longer satisfied the clinicians. It seemed better to remain vague than to embrace doctrines that appeared clearly inadequate.

Well into the nineteenth century, this view prevailed among leading clinicians. William Pultney Alison (1790–1859), an outstanding clinician at Edinburgh, declared that "the first important step in medical science is the separation of the phenomena of the living body from all those which are comprised in the science of Chemistry and Mechanics."[6]

The "action of the vessels," an essentially vitalistic concept, applied to topics other than inflammation. It was used especially to explain secretion. Many different secretions had their origin in the blood. The existence of secretory cells was not known, and many functions now attributed to cells were then ascribed to the capillary wall. Numerous contemporary theories have been well summarized by John Bostock and by Robley Dunglison.[7]

For Cullen "the action of the vessels of the secretory organs has a considerable share in determining both the quantity and quality of the secreted fluid."[8] Something was happening at the site of the minute vessels, but he did not know what. Despite the vast amount of experimental work since Cullen wrote, and the existence of chemical theories of secretion, Bostock said that "we must conceive

of it [secretion] as originating in *the vital action of the vessels,*
which enables them to transmit the blood, or certain parts of it, to
the various organs."[9]

EXPERIMENTAL STUDIES

Between 1801 and 1804, A. P. Wilson Philip (1770?–1851) published *A Treatise of Febrile Diseases,* of which an American edition
appeared in 1816.[10] He denied that inflammation consisted of increased action of the local vessels. Action meant a muscular contraction of the vessel wall that narrowed the lumen. Inflammation,
however, involved a localized accumulation of blood. How could
increased action lead to accumulation of blood? As an explanation,
he postulated two types of force, one tending to dilatation of the
vessels, the other offering a resistance to dilatation.

The forward impulse of the blood, derived from the contraction
of the heart and the larger arteries, he called the *vis à tergo.*
This, a distending force directed peripherally, acted against the
resistance furnished by the musculoelastic structure of the smaller
vessels. The normal balance between these forces might be vari-
ously disturbed. If, for example, the *vis à tergo* increased and the
powers of resistance inherent in the vessels remained the same, or
if the latter were weakened and the *vis à tergo* remained the
same, then "the vessel must suffer a morbid degree of dilatation."[11]
Inflammation depended on the relations between the distending
and the resisting forces.

In an inflamed part, "the capillary arteries [sic] are in a state of
debility, the larger in that of increased excitement" (ibid., p. 32). A
diminished action of the capillaries resulted in dilatation. The larger
vessels, in contrast, had an increased action and were contracted.
The inflammatory process would terminate when the force of the
capillaries regained a due proportion to the *vis à tergo.* Inflammation could thus be cured by increasing the action of the capillaries
or diminishing that of the larger arteries. Increased action of *all*
the vessels did not result in inflammation (p. 45).

These views Philip derived from experiments on living tissues.
The web of a frog's foot, the tail of a fish, and the mesentery of a
rabbit could be subjected to direct microscopic examination, even
with the imperfect instruments of the day. He could directly observe
that the small vessels and the larger vessels could show opposite

types of change. He described his experiments in detail and provided illustrative drawings of successive stages in the process (pp. 43–53).

His theory of inflammation modified that of Cullen. A debility was induced in the capillaries, and "to correct this morbid state" the larger vessels of the part were excited to increased action. This increased the *vis à tergo*. This latter force was a principal causal factor, since "inflammation may arise either from a debility of the capillaries, or an increased *vis à tergo*" (pp. 71–73). Philip's discussion and his evidence point out the difference between the armchair theorizing of Cullen and actual experimental work. It illustrates with special clarity some differences between eighteenth-century thinking and that of the nineteenth century.

CULLEN'S CLASSIFICATION OF FEVERS

When we pass from the study of inflammation to the study of fevers, we encounter a new type of problem, involving classification. Medical scientists are not content merely to observe and treat individual cases but must also bring order into clinical experience. To do this, they separate cases into kinds or classes, each showing certain distinguishing and identifying marks. They can then arrange these groups or categories into the more inclusive and the less inclusive.

A large group may be subdivided into progressively smaller groups. Such a hierarchical arrangement comprises formal classification, which, when applied to diseases, is called a nosology. The various levels of subdivision have technical names, which can be rather confusing. At present, I will discuss only one group of diseases and the definitions that characterize them, namely, the febrile disorders.

For the entire all-inclusive group of febrile diseases, Cullen gave a succinct definition or characterization. All fever cases could be identified by the presence of certain symptoms: a chill or a chilly feeling, a rapid pulse, increased body temperature, and a disinclination to movement (or, in a more literal translation of the Latin, "a diminished strength, especially of the limbs").[12]

This large and rather vague category Cullen named *pyrexiae* (fevers), which he subdivided into five subordinate and more sharply differentiated groups. These all shared the features that defined the *pyrexiae,* but in addition each had its own special character, supposedly unique to itself.

One subgroup he called *phlegmasiae,* in which the distinguishing feature was some localized inflammation, coupled with impairment of function. The individual diseases thus characterized were named according to the organ involved, such as ophthalmia, hepatitis, cystitis, arthritis, and the like. We recall Cullen's dictum, that a local inflammation, if intense enough, would lead to fever. The inflammation would presumably be primary, the fever, secondary.

Another subdivision, the exanthemata, was identified by a skin eruption, as in smallpox, measles, or scarlatina. In a further subgroup, the *hemorrhagiae,* he placed the febrile conditions accompanied by hemorrhage. This feature was the common thread that united such diseases as phthisis ("consumption," or tuberculosis), hemorrhoids, and menorrhagia. Correlative, in a sense, with this group was the next, the *profluviae,* a word commonly translated as fluxes. Here the characteristic mark, the defining feature, was an increased secretion that was not bloody, such as catarrh and dysentery. We can see a residue of old humoral concepts, with one group of diseases characterized by a flow of blood, another by a flow of serous humor.

The remaining subclass (which in his exposition Cullen discussed first), he called *febres,* fever in the strict sense. In this class he placed the diseases that had the signs of fever (*pyrexiae*) but without any primary local disease. Such fevers were regarded as primary, or essential (or, in a later terminology, idiopathic). They were considered to be general, affecting the whole system, without any clear point of attack or localizing features.

In this classification, the English word *fever* occurs in two different contexts, as a large and all-inclusive class, the *pyrexiae,* and also as a subordinate and more sharply differentiated subclass, the *febres.* In Latin, *pyrexiae* is distinct from *febres,* but the English word *fever* remains the same in the two distinct usages. Much confusion has resulted, especially from writers who, when they discussed the causes of fevers, have not always been clear which group they were talking about.

The concepts of fever expanded markedly in the nineteenth century. To appreciate the progressive changes, we must have a firm grasp on Cullen's views, which dominated medical theory at the end of the eighteenth century. In his presentation, Cullen subdivided the category *febres,* the essential or primary fevers, into two groups, according to their temporal course. One group he called intermittent fevers, the other, continued fevers. The intermittents (including our malaria) showed recurrent paroxysms but, in the intervals, a freedom from symptoms. Continued fevers ran a more or less uninterrupted course. Even though some partial remissions might occur, there was no full intermission.

The entire group of continued fever, under various names, had already received substantial attention from earlier writers. Some of the earlier literature I have noted in my *Medical World of the Eighteenth Century,* but there is fuller coverage in the more recent writings of William Bynum and Dale Smith.[13]

Cullen dealt with three major problems. First, What is a fever? The answer tried to identify the essential nature, that is, the proximal cause. Second, What factors induce a fever; or differently phrased, What are the remote causes? And third, By what steps did the remote cause or causes actually produce the fever? Differently expressed, What is the pathogenesis? Cullen's answers typified the thought modes of the eighteenth century. Successive innovations, offered by different authors, reveal the slow transformations of medical thinking.

In analyzing the overall nature of fever, Cullen first gave a rather detailed account of the clinical phenomena. The paroxysm of intermittent fever seemed to offer a clear example that could be generalized for all fevers. He noted the initial stage of languor, followed by a sensation of cold, which may progress to a shaking chill or rigor. This is followed by the hot stage, increased body heat, which, if the patient survives, persists until the sweating stage. With the onset of sweating, the paroxysm terminates. In different fevers, the paroxysms differ in degree and in circumstances.[14] All febrile conditions, he thought, had a basically similar course.

Then, to explain the phenomena, he had to indicate the proximal cause and the pathogenesis and show how each major component developed. In expounding the proximal cause, Cullen did not provide any direct empirical evidence, let alone any experimental demonstration. He offered only chains of reasoning and inferences, linked together by conceptual entities—hypotheses.

Cullen assumed that each stage of the fever induced the next, in a chainlike connection. The cold stage "is always preceded by strong marks of a general debility prevailing in the system" (ibid., par. 35). The debility, however it came into being would entail the cold stage, which in turn led to the hot stage, and this to the sweating stage. Whatever induced the debility would thus set in motion the entire chainlike process.

He expounded his views in considerable detail (pars. 53–57). The initial phenomenon, debility, acted first on the brain, reducing its level of energy. This reduced energy, corresponding to clinical languor, altered the tone of the "extreme vessels," to produce in them an atony. Then there occurred a compensatory physiological reaction, attributed to the *vis medicatrix naturae*, or healing power of nature, that tried to restore equilibrium. The compensatory reaction took the form of a spasm of the extreme vessels, especially on the surface of the body. This spasm corresponded to the clinical cold stage.

As the next sequential step, the spasm in the very small vessels "proves an irritation to the heart and arteries" (par. 41), resulting in their increased action. This was the physiological equivalent of the hot stage. The spasm continued until it was relaxed or overcome by the increased action. When relaxation took place, the normal tonus of the vessels was restored, the sweating stage occurred, and the patient was on the way to recovery.

To an unsympathetic modern reader all this may sound silly. Nevertheless, a close reading of the text induces a great admiration for Cullen's acumen and his critical sense. He had little physiological information at his disposal, but the information he did have he integrated with clinical observations. He used the only tools at his command—analogy and comparison, inference, and reliance on widely accepted concepts.

In addition he had a striking critical attitude and made a definite effort to avoid dogmatism. Quite often he used expressions such as "It seems to me probable that," or the equivalent. Also worthy of mention is his discussion of alternate schemata of pathogenesis, such as the idea that fever resulted from the introduction of noxious matter into the body, with resulting efforts to eliminate it (pars. 49–50).

At the same time, he was hobbled by the modes of thinking that pervaded his entire era—the passion for comprehensive explanation, the reliance on logical inference without any empirical confirmation, and the facile generalization from one or two instances. Although Cullen was systematic in his theories, he was not systematic in his approach to empirical data. He was not in any sense an empirical investigator. We shall see how all these characteristics gradually became less prominent in the course of a century—although, be it stated parenthetically, they have by no means disappeared even today.

The proximal cause of all fever, for Cullen, was a single pattern of physiological changes, whose stages might vary in intensity and duration. From clinical observation, physicians noted different kinds of fever. If there were only a single uniform proximal cause, how to explain the clinical diversity? The answers lay not with the proximal cause but with variations in the remote causes.

Cullen made explicit the clinical features of the two main types of essential fevers, the intermittent and the continued. Intermittent fevers (our clinical malaria), with their characteristic clinical course, seemed straightforward enough. The chief difficulties lay with the continued fevers.

Two principal forms of continued fevers had long been distinguished, under a variety of names, of which the most general were inflammatory fever and nervous fever. In the former the pulse was strong and the bodily reactions vigorous. To this type Cullen offered his own nomenclature, *synocha*. This he characterized as having a strong rapid pulse, with no disturbance of the sensory functions. For this disease, bloodletting was the appropriate remedy.

To the second main type, the "nervous" or "low nervous" fever, he gave the name *typhus*. It showed a weak pulse, a prostration and loss of bodily strength, and severely disturbed sensorium. Bloodletting was generally not advisable. Then he opened a Pandora's box by distinguishing a third type, *synochus,* that started out as a synocha and ended as a typhus. He was asserting that one kind, supposedly distinct, would transform into another kind, equally distinct. He noted further that the category typhus probably included several subgroups, "not yet well ascertained by observation" (par. 70).

To explain the diversity, Cullen invoked different remote causes, all of which, by inducing an initial debility, could entail the same proximal cause. The initial debility then brought about the rest of the sequence composing the fever.

Cullen discussed the remote causes of the major diseases under three principal heads. A *contagion* was the actual material agent that would transfer a disease, such as smallpox, from one person to another. The transmission took place through contact, direct or indirect, between a sick person and a healthy person. When this took place, the disease was contagious.

Miasma, on the other hand, whose synonym was malaria, or bad air, was the exhalation from swamps that induced intermittent fevers. This agent could not spread by direct contact between the sick and healthy. Hence, intermittent fevers were not contagious.

A third major remote cause involved various environmental features, of which *cold* was perhaps the most important, but which also included such factors as bad food and fatigue. The complexities inherent in these remote causes will emerge in the course of this book. Suffice it now to mention them as factors contributing to the diversity of fevers.

Cullen's explanations gave only the illusion of precision. His definitions, reflecting the available relevant data, were quite vague. The real nature of a "disease entity" was unclear, and for most diseases the adequacy of his definitions was subject to dispute. Real precision could not emerge until vastly more data were available. This increase in knowledge occurred slowly and with much controversy.

I would note here some problems lurking in Cullen's exposition. How did inflammation link up with fever? Can one kind of fever really transform into another, or does each clinical type have a fixity, a specificity of some sort? How secure are the assertions regarding the proximal cause of fever? Or regarding the pathogenesis of fevers? What is a disease entity? Do clinical differences indicate distinct entities or only varieties of a single entity? And above all, how can we be sure?

Cullen himself was not troubled by these problems. The difficulties became apparent only gradually, as nineteenth-century physicians uncovered new data or had new ideas, which in turn led them into new modes of thinking.

BENJAMIN RUSH, AN EIGHTEENTH-CENTURY THINKER

At the beginning of the nineteenth century, Benjamin Rush was the outstanding American physician. With unusual intellectual endowment and a medical training excellent for its period, he had absorbed the medical concepts current in Great Britain and then, with some modifications, transplanted them into the United States. A thoroughly eighteenth-century figure, he did not embody the emerging nineteenth-century ideas.

At the age of fourteen he graduated from what later became Princeton College and then, for almost six years, served an apprenticeship with the leading practitioner in Philadelphia. For further training it was necessary to go abroad. He spent two years in Edinburgh, earning his M.D. degree in 1766, and then devoted more than a year to further study in London and Paris.

Before he left Philadelphia, he was being groomed for the chair of chemistry in the new medical school that John Morgan (1735–89) would establish in Philadelphia.[15] On his return to the United States, Rush was elected professor of chemistry. Competent scholars have called him "the founder of American chemistry."[16] In 1789, on the death of Morgan, Rush was appointed professor of the theory and practice of physic. Through his extensive lecturing and writing he greatly influenced medical practice as well as theory. Some of his students, becoming teachers in their turn, helped to spread his influence, as formal medical education spread westward.

Rush, who achieved prominence in many fields, has been the subject of much biographical study.[17] I shall pass over his political and sociological activities and deal only with his doctrine of fevers. In this regard, while his passion for bloodletting has attracted popular interest, little attention has been paid to his specifically medical concepts.[18]

While abroad, Rush absorbed the ideas of John Brown, once a pupil of Cullen, who modified his master's teachings into a remarkable system.[19] Brown offered a highly simplistic theory that could explain all medical phenomena by ignoring any discordant data. He reduced physiology to two components. *Excitability* meant the capacity of an organism to respond to stimulus. It was the potentiality of reaction. Correlative to this was *excitement*, referring to the reaction itself, as the potential became actual.

Health depended on the balance between the capacity to react and the concrete activity itself. An imbalance would constitute debility, which existed in two distinct forms. One type, indirect debility, would be induced by excessive excitement (i.e., activity). On the other hand, not enough excitement (insufficient reaction) would produce the opposite disease, direct debility. The physician had to decide whether the debility was direct or indirect and make the correction through appropriate therapy. In cases of insufficient excitement, the proper treatment was stimulation. If excitement were excessive, treatment was sedation.

Unfortunately, sometimes the same clinical appearance might result from either excess or deficiency of excitement. Some modern examples might make this a little clearer: too much exercise can produce debility, with lessened capacity for further reaction, but too little exercise can also reduce the capacity to react. Again, too much food can lead to repletion and loss of energy (debility), but insufficient food will also induce debility. We can readily assert that excess and deficiency can both produce the "same" effect, provided we ignore all the differences.

With some change of nomenclature, Rush adopted these features of Brown's system. Fevers that showed an excess of excitement corresponded, more or less, with the synocha of Cullen, or inflammatory fever. Debility from too little excitement corresponded roughly to the low nervous fevers of eighteenth-century authors, which Cullen designated as typhus. Factors that contributed to overabundance of stimuli included heat, intemperance, excessive exercise, and violent emotion ("stimulating passions of the mind"). Too little excitement might result from "debilitating passions," cold, excessive evacuations, and inadequate nutrition.[20]

These were all contingent factors, which might or might not induce a fever. Rush, however, sought the feature that was present in every case and necessarily produced fever. Exposure to cold, for example, often regarded as a causal agent, might or might not produce disease. This inconsistency might, in turn, depend on other factors, such as predisposition or unusual susceptibility.

Another condition that might or might not lead to fever he called the "forming state." This could affect the whole system, with weakness of the limbs, fatigue, chilliness, and other manifestations. Today we would regard all this as a prodromal phase of an infection. Rush, however, thought differently. These reactions did not necessarily lead into the florid manifestations that constituted fever, as he understood it. Instead, by rest, or "gentle remedies," the symptoms might be "dissipated" and the patient recover with no further disturbance.

These early stages of indisposition might pass off without further manifestation and no "fever" result. Hence they did not compose *the* cause, which for Rush involved necessity. Rush wanted to identify the feature that necessarily and inevitably led to fever and would constitute its proximal cause. As such it would, according to its "greater or less force and extent," correlate with the different degrees of fever. This reaction, he asserted without direct evidence, was essentially "of a convulsive nature . . . situated primarily in the blood vessels, and particularly in the arteries" (ibid., p. 9).

For Rush, then, fever consisted of "morbid excitement" of the blood vessels. This, the proximal cause of fever, was "convulsive" in nature. It could vary in different parts of the body and affect the vascular system in different ways. The arteries of one part need not respond in the same way as those of another part, and at any given moment the heart need not react in the same sense as did the arteries. "The arteries in the head, lungs, and abdominal viscera are sometimes excited in a high degree while the arteries in the extremities exhibit marks of a feeble morbid action." And he gave other examples of localized action in one place, coinciding with its absence elsewhere (pp. 10, 11).

Such morbid activity, he thought, might overtake the blood vessels as a result of stimuli that normally might have no effect. In a state of debility, a small stimulus could have profound effects. If a convulsive action of blood vessels were induced, then fever would result. He gave as an example the (alleged) observation that, soon after vigorous exercise (with its subsequent debility), a person might come down with a fever (p. 13).

The proximal cause of fever, then, was a convulsive action of the blood vessels. There is no need to follow Rush in detail as he gave various examples and organized them into a coherent doctrine. He explained away every apparent exception. He offered a systematic account of fevers, consonant with the principles of Cullen, but differing in details. Convulsive action, along with excitability and excitement, debility, forming stage, and predisposition, composed the vocabulary by which he explained fever.

He did not perceive the gaps in his logic, nor the merely verbal character of his explanation. His assertions had little grounding in concrete observation. Today, these views might seem strange indeed, but Rush cannot be judged by today's standards. For him, fever was whatever fitted his definition. What did not fit was not a fever. We are reminded, perhaps, of the rhyme about Benjamin Jowett, the great Oxford scholar:

My name is Benjamin Jowett
I'm the master of this college.
If there is anything to know, I know it,
What I don't know is not knowledge.

With Rush, there was but one fever, whose cause he dogmatically asserted. Clinical variation had usually been attributed to different remote causes, but Rush had little interest in remote causes. The significant feature, for him, was the uniform proximate cause, namely, the convulsive reaction of the blood vessels that occurred in all fevers.

THE UNITY AND DIVERSITY OF FEVERS

Rush thought in simplistic fashion. If all fevers had the same proximal cause, then the subsidiary and inconstant remote factors were of no great importance. As an illustration of this thinking, I would point to a death certificate, which supposedly gives the cause of death. Rush, I suggest, might have been perfectly content to put, in every case, "cardiac arrest." Death implied the presence of that cause, and the presence of the cause implied death. The equivalence is necessary, by virtue of the definition.

In fevers, the unity of the (proximal) cause led Rush to an analogy in which he compared fever to fire. "Thus, fire is a unit, whether it be produced by friction, percussion, electricity, fermentation, or by a piece of wood or coal in a state of inflammation." Just as fire was a unit, so too was fever (pp. 15–17). The single proximate cause, the convulsive action of the blood vessels, placed all febrile conditions into a single group.

Still, there seemed to be differences among fevers. In trying to explain the appearance of diversity, Rush collided with the current views of nosology. Nosologists classified fevers in a fashion similar to that used for plants or animals. Rush strongly opposed any such analysis. Plants and animals, he thought, had unchanging characteristics—diseases did not. "The oak tree and the lion possess exactly the same properties which they did nearly 6,000 years ago. But who can say the same thing of any one disease?" Diseases, he thought, were intermingled and passed one into another. "The pulmonary consumption is sometimes transformed into the head-ach, rheumatism, diarrhea, and mania, in the course of two or three months. . . . The bilious fever often appears in the same person in the form of colic, dysentery, inflammation of the liver, lungs, and brain, in the course of five or six days."

Then, too, the lion had not imparted his specific qualities to any other animal, but not so with diseases. "Phrenitis, gastritis, enteritis, nephritis, and rheumatism all appear at the same time in the gout and yellow fever." Diseases, for Rush, had a fluid character, with none of the sharp demarcations that characterized plants or animals. Nosology, he thought, depends on separations that were artificial and false. It erects "imaginary boundaries between things which are of a homogeneous nature" (pp. 33–34).

The problem has a deeper foundation, namely, the question, What is a disease? Is it a thing, an entity, a material object, a series of relationships, a pattern, a set of physiological reactions? Later in the nineteenth century, the concept of ontology denied that a disease was a real entity. The problem goes back to medieval disputes between nominalists and realists. Even today, the dispute is still active, with the not infrequent assertion, There are no diseases, only sick patients.[21]

Rush pointed to a feature common to all fevers, namely, the "morbid action or excitement in some part of the body. Its different seats and degrees should no more be multiplied into different diseases than the numerous and different effects of heat and light upon our globe should be multiplied into a plurality of suns."[22]

While all fevers depended on a single cause, namely, a "morbid action in the blood vessels," this action could vary in force, frequency, or the locus of its activity. Rush used these distinctions to explain the clinical diversities of fevers and inflammation (ibid., p. 57).

He divided fevers into two groups. In one, the entire system was affected, without localized changes; in the other, a localized inflammation also occurred. He distinguished "states" of fever. These were not separate diseases but varieties of the single condition, fever. The different states could succeed one another and readily change one into another. There were twelve "primary" states, from which many others were "compounded."

One example of primary states is the synocha, or "common inflammatory state of fever," which attacked suddenly, with chills, a rapid, tense pulse, a great thirst, and pains in bones and joints, as well as other regions. If of lesser intensity, this state was a synocula. The typhus state showed great debility, "accompanied for the most part by feeble excitement in the blood-vessels from a feeble stimulus" (p. 48). It was, in a sense, the opposite of the synocha. Especially confusing was the typhoid state, to be discussed in later chapters.

Rush had so far described "general" fever, which affected primarily the whole arterial system with but little local disease. He also discussed the combinations of general and local states, where a particular organ or system was primarily affected. Examples were the intestinal, the pulmonary, the rheumatic, and the arthritic states of fever. Of special interest was the cephalic state, which included "the phrenitic, lethargic, apoplectic, paralytic, hydrocephalic, and maniacal states of fever." He emphasized that "madness is originally a state of fever." Its causes, he thought, were the same as those that induced other states of fever. In the brains of "maniacs" were found the same phenomena "exhibited by other inflamed viscera after death . . . effusions . . . abscesses, and schirrhus. . . . Madness," he said, "is as much an original disease of the blood vessels, as any other state of fever." A deranged mind, "is the effect only of chronic inflammation of the brain" (pp. 56–57).

We might well ask ourselves, What is the difference between a "disease" and "state"? Rush did not provide a satisfactory answer. He drove the concept of separate diseases out the door, but they slipped back through the window.

In 1791 he declared, "We live, gentlemen, in a revolutionary age. Our science has caught the spirit of the times, and more improvements have been made in all its branches within the last twenty years than had been made in a century before."[23] Rush, lacking flexibility, did not really understand the changes taking place around him. Turning resolutely toward the past, he made verbal elaborations that led nowhere. Fixed ideas limited his thinking, and he rejected anything that might seem discordant. He had placed all fevers on a truly Procrustean bed and then, through verbal manipulation, made everything fit. Nevertheless, as we shall see, he did raise questions that have not been fully answered even today.

EMPHASIS ON THE NERVOUS SYSTEM

Toward the end of the eighteenth century, changing concepts and methods were slowly exerting their influence, especially in France and, to a lesser extent, in Great Britain. These changes were relatively slow in crossing the Atlantic. Benjamin Rush, for example, was not affected by the new intellectual currents of the 1790s, and not until the 1820s did the new spirit effect much change in American medicine. Meanwhile, however, European writers were showing a mixture of the old and the new. Henry Clutterbuck (1767–1856), twenty years younger than Rush, also remained quite steadfast in what I call eighteenth-century thought modes.

Clutterbuck elaborated the old concepts and did not react to the new. He trained as a surgeon through the usual apprenticeship, and later obtained the M.D. degree, in 1804. In 1807 he published *An Inquiry into the Seat and Nature of Fever*. A monograph, *An Essay on Pyrexia,* appeared in 1837 and was reprinted in Philadelphia the next year.[24] When he wrote his first book, he had relatively little practical experience and drew his data chiefly from the works of other writers. His doctrine, he said, represented "a fair and legitimate deduction from generally admitted facts . . . strongly supported by analogy." He provided a tissue of inferences drawn from "accepted facts"—which others had provided. At first glance, the insistence on facts might seem a part of the developing empirical influence of the early nineteenth century. Clutterbuck, however, ignored the crucial feature of the enlightened empiricism:

he was not critical of the alleged evidence. He did not ask, Is it really so? Is it really so?

In the eighteenth-century there had been pressure to find a single comprehensive explanation for the phenomena of disease. Cullen, wanting to unify his doctrine of fevers, laid great stress on activity of the nervous system. Clutterbuck expanded this view. Thus, the stomach had been suggested as the primary seat of fever. Clutterbuck thought such an origin improbable. Gastric disturbance, he believed, would be secondary to a more basic source, which he placed in a "disordered state of the brain."[25] In fever, he pointed out, the functions of the brain never fail to be "perverted" in some way. Without denying the importance of the stomach in fevers, he considered a disturbance of the brain as still more primary.

He pointed to various factors that had been considered remote causes of fever, such as heat, cold, intemperance, irritations, improper foods, miasmata, contagions, poisons of various kinds. Although for some of these the modes of action were obscure, others "are known to exert their action chiefly on the brain and nervous system" (ibid., p. 86). Then he made an enormous jump: that to produce a general (rather than a merely local) effect, irritation "must operate through the medium of the brain" (p. 89). It was, he thought, "at least probable, that the brain is the chief and primary seat of fever" (p. 97) and that disturbance in the brain function "is the source of the principal phenomena, or pathognomonic symptoms." The disturbance, he thought, "is either a state of actual inflammation, or, at least, a condition nearly allied to it" (pp. 99–100).

Clutterbuck's belief rested on indirect evidence, namely, the presence of disturbed cerebral function. As we have seen, Cullen regarded altered function, combined with pain, as the chief evidence of internal inflammation. Clutterbuck fell victim to a simple logical fallacy. Inflammation led to disturbance of function. Therefore, a disturbed function was a sign of inflammation. He concluded that fever, with its clouding of the sensorium, consisted in a "topical inflammation of the brain" but admitted that the arguments "derived principally from analogy" (p. 146).

We today might think that anatomical dissection would provide evidence to settle the question one way or the other, whether inflammation was or was not present. However, such a direct recourse to experience was not possible in the early nineteenth century. No one could distinguish inflammation from congestion, and a congestion noted at autopsy was readily called inflammation. There were no techniques for microscopic study of the brain. All conclusions had to rest solely on gross observation of autopsy material. Clutterbuck admitted that "the evidence furnished by dissection is not absolutely conclusive."

His reasoning is interesting (see pp. 156–163). The very nature of the brain, he said, renders it unsuitable for "accurate examination," so that our knowledge of it is "exceedingly limited." Because the brain has a tendency to "decomposition" (i.e., postmortem changes), we have little acquaintance with its "sound and natural appearance." Hence, published descriptions regarding the state of the brain are "perhaps little to be relied on." We cannot really tell whether any changes that might be described in the literature "are the effects of disease, or of a beginning decomposition of parts" (i.e., whether disease or artifact). Furthermore, all too often the brain was not examined at autopsy, and even when it was, the examiners might not be "perfectly competent to the task." Moreover, subtle changes may have occurred in the brain that were not "manifested to the senses." The failure to find changes did not mean that changes did not exist.

Clutterbuck concluded that morbid anatomy did not give reliable evidence concerning inflammation in the brain. All his reasons formed an interlocking whole: Changes might be so slight that they defied detection with present means. If changes were found, they might represent postmortem artifacts. However, since the brain was not often examined, and since the examiners were often not skilled or reliable, we do not know whether changes really existed or not.

The overall lack of empirical evidence did not disturb him. He maintained that "the medullary substance of the brain is the primary seat of morbid affection in fever" (p. 158). This, admittedly a "supposition," he justified by the disturbance of function. While admitting his reliance on remote analogies, he nevertheless asserted forcefully, "The conclusion appears to me irrefutable:—that the symptoms of fever are the symptoms of inflamed brain, and that the latter is the immediate cause of the former; or rather, that fever and inflammation of the brain are identical affections" (p. 178). Cerebral inflammation would be the proximate cause of fever: the terms were interchangeable.

Fever was not a "disease of the whole system," as was commonly supposed, but actually *"a topical affection of the brain"* (p. 421). The febrile state was merely symptomatic of this brain affection. But if all fever were symptomatic (that is, secondary to an inflammation), then there was no such entity as an essential or idiopathic fever. This view made a considerable appeal through the 1820s.

Clutterbuck was, in a sense, the acme of eighteenth-century rationalism. He started with alleged facts, which he accepted uncritically. By verbal manipulation that he considered logical, he arrived at conclusions that he asserted dogmatically. He did nothing to enlarge the data base on which his concepts rested, and he did not support his inferences with empirical demonstration. He was untouched by the new critical empiricism.

BROUSSAIS AND "PHYSIOLOGICAL MEDICINE"

Clutterbuck's methodology correlated well with the influential doctrines of French physician François Joseph Victor Broussais. Broussais first studied medicine with his father, a country surgeon in Brittany. From his twentieth to his twenty-fifth years, he was a naval surgeon. Highly ambitious, he went to Paris in 1800 to get a medical degree and fell under the influence of Bichat and the remarkable group of physicians active in Paris at that time.[26] After receiving his degree in 1803, he had a long period of military service with the imperial armies of Napoleon. He was essentially a man of practice, who nevertheless tried to theorize in the new mode.

A prolific and disputatious writer, Broussais constantly engaged in polemics and wordy expositions. His first major work, in 1808, laid the groundwork for his doctrines, elaborated in an even more important work of 1816, and in later studies. His concepts had only a modest American audience until translations were published in Philadelphia between 1828 and 1832.[27]

Broussais was primarily a clinician exposed to the new ideas emerging at the end of the eighteenth century. The new French influence manifested itself in detailed clinicopathological correlations. Hospitals were large, and eager clinicians performed vast numbers of autopsies, correlating their findings with the clinical data. Through this method, in the early nineteenth century French clinicians greatly enlarged the knowledge of pulmonary diseases and fevers. I discuss these advances in greater detail in chapter 5.

Broussais's early training was very much in the old mode. However, when he became a disciple of Bichat, he learned the need for analysis—the reduction of a whole into its component parts. Broussais applied the concept by stressing the role of individual organs in disease. His extensive autopsy experience provided a great quantity of data, but in his interpretations he was extremely uncritical, wordy, and dogmatic. He tried to explain disease through basic physiological processes taking place in the individual organs. Such an attitude he called physiological medicine and claimed it as peculiarly his own. So loud and frequent were his claims that most subsequent writers have accepted them at face value.

Physicians, however, even though they may not have stressed individual organs, have always explained their observations through the physiological principles prevailing at that time. Galen had analyzed diseases in physiological terms as he conceived them. When Galenism declined, the genesis and course of disease were explained in different functional terms. Cullen, a modest and effective eclectic, propounded physiological theories, as did his much less modest pupil John Brown. All of this was physiological medicine.

Broussais, too, explained disease by principles he accepted as physiological truths. His basic concept was vitality, that is, the aggregate of properties that distinguished the living from the nonliving. To perform their function, the organs must "enjoy the degree of vitality necessary for the proper execution of the function."[28] The word *proper*, however, remained entirely undefined. The vitality of particular organs might become "exalted" or "diminished," as they exhibited greater (or less) functional activity; but the changes were primarily local and might or might not spread to other organs (ibid., prop. 283).

Broussais manipulated words without giving them much content. An exalted vitality meant "an action, resulting from modifying stimulants, superior to that which maintains health." Health was a balance, and if the stimuli exceed those found in health, disease would result. Such a "superexcitation" (i.e., irritation) led to a morbid congestion. The terms *irritation* and *congestion* defined each other with complete circularity. Irritation induced congestion, and congestion results from irritation. Furthermore, irritation, if sufficiently intense, would lead to inflammation. Words were chasing themselves around in vague circles, and they remained isolated from concrete evidence (props. 77, 83, 99).

BROUSSAIS AND "SYMPATHY"

All these terms he integrated through the concept of sympathy, wherein a disturbance in one part produced a related disturbance in a different part. The disturbance might involve the functional activity, or the anatomical change he called inflammation, or both. This transfer of irritation, effected by sympathy, occurred via the nervous system.

New studies in anatomy clearly distinguished two parts of the nervous system. The great sympathetic nerve, controlling the visceral functions, mediated the "organic" sympathies. Sensation and voluntary movement, however, were mediated by the cerebrospinal axis (brain, spinal cord, and peripheral nerves). This central nervous system was responsible for "sympathies of relation." The two parts were connected and each could affect the other.

These concepts Broussais used to explain the relations of inflammation and fever. All physiological actions were attributed to excitation. When this passed beyond the normal stage, it became an irritation and, if severe enough, an inflammation. Slight irritation would affect sympathetically only the immediately adjacent tissues; if more intense, it would spread to affect the nervous system more widely (prop. 86). Through sympathy, inflammation could thus spread by way of the nervous system. Broussais used a single set of concepts to explain neurophysiological reactions, the spread of inflammation, and also the origins of fever.

When an irritation involved the heart, fever resulted, with its quickened pulse and increased heat. The spread of irritation ordinarily would follow either organic sympathies or sympathies of relation, but a crossover, via nerve pathways, could readily take place. An irritation once transmitted to the brain could then be "reflected" into other organs. Usually the brain would reflect irritations to the locomotor and sensory systems but, if intensity were strong, could also affect the stomach through the sympathetic nerve. Broussais declared, "it is through the medium of the brain that the heart and stomach receive the irritation from a focus of inflammation developed elsewhere than in these three organs" (prop. 113).

In sympathetic reactions there was no proportionality between cause and effect. Organs sympathetically affected might "contract a degree of irritation greater than that of the organ from which they derive their irritation." The duration and intensity of irritation were determined by "idiosyncrasy" and "modifying agents," unspecified. Anything unusual was explained away by "idiosyncracy" (prop. 97).

If through the process of sympathy an inflammation anywhere were intense enough to reach first the brain or stomach and then the heart, fever would result. Irritations that spread in this way need not give symptoms pointing to the site of origin. A small initial irritation, of which the patient was not aware, might produce an intense sympathetic reaction. Involvement of the stomach (or gastrointestinal tract), even without any direct symptoms, could thus cause a fever through sympathetic spread (props. 136–38).

This doctrine led to a necessary inference: all fevers were secondary or symptomatic and belonged to the category that Cullen had named *phlegmasiae*. There were no primary fevers. What other physicians regarded as "essential" fevers were all referable to hidden inflammation, ordinarily some form of gastroenteritis. This concept "explained" diseases such as bilious, gastric, mucous, adynamic, or putrid fevers, as well as yellow fever or typhus or even synochus (prop. 137; See also props. 138–42).

But what was the evidence? Broussais maintained that his inferences were empirically based, and he rested his conclusions on his autopsy findings. He claimed to have actually observed the inflammations that were not clinically apparent. Autopsies showed marks of inflammation "almost universally, in the mucous membranes of the alimentary canal," and this change had been accorded a causal role.

John Eberle (1788–1838), a contemporary American physician, pointed out some defects. The observed changes could be a consequence of the fever rather than the cause. Moreover, inflammation was often diagnosed merely from the reddened appearance of the mucosa. This might be only postmortem change, an artifact, not a symptom of disease.[29]

Broussais had no greater knowledge about inflammation than had Clutterbuck, but he expanded his ignorance to a much greater degree. He evolved a complex schema of sympathy and of hypothetical action to support his claim, namely, that all fevers, without exception, were secondary to inflammation, somewhere. Even if no focus was manifest clinically, the fever could always be considered secondary to a gastroenteritis. If there were an autopsy, Broussais could always "prove" his point by finding "inflammation" somewhere. Without an autopsy, he postulated its existence. When he lacked concrete evidence, he created ad hoc hypotheses to fill the gap. Broussais remained essentially an eighteenth-century physician, with the eighteenth-century passion for a comprehensive system. He was a systematist, ambitious beyond his intellectual capacity.

Inadequate knowledge of inflammation was the weakest link in theories of the day. Only later in the nineteenth century, with emergence of cell theory and improved microscopic study, and still later, with the discovery of bacteria, would the nature of inflammation, and its relations to fever, have a sound foundation.

AMERICAN RECIDIVISM: CHARLES CALDWELL

In the early nineteenth century, Clutterbuck represented a reactionary British viewpoint that ignored the newer medical trends slowly becoming influential. In the United States we have an excellent example of that same attitude, which resolutely looked backward instead of forward. Charles Caldwell (1772–1853) exemplified this trend. He played a considerable role in the development of American medicine and exerted a quite unfortunate effect on medical education.

His autobiography, a minor classic in American medical literature, reveals him as an egomaniac and a braggart.[30] Well educated as a youth, he began to study medicine as an apprentice. Dissatisfied with the teaching he received, he soon left his preceptor to attend the medical school in Philadelphia, where he absorbed Edinburgh doctrines filtered through Benjamin Rush. Graduating in 1796, Caldwell practiced in Philadelphia until 1819. Then, after failing to win the professorship of medicine, he left Philadelphia for Transylvania University in Lexington, Kentucky. The rest of his long and active life he spent in Kentucky, first at Lexington and then at Louisville.

Ohio and Kentucky were then the cultural outposts of the West, where newly established medical schools trained large numbers of medical practitioners. Caldwell's dogmatic and reactionary teachings, apparently well received in the new medical schools, tended to block the diffusion of newer trends that were, by that time, gaining a foothold in the eastern states.

Caldwell's monograph, *An Analysis of Fever,* published in 1825, gives us a fine insight into the teaching that he offered his students.[31] In large part he more or less echoed Cullen. A "morbid impression," he said, initiated the febrile process. Then came the stage of "access" (our prodromal state); then the chill or cold stage, succeeded by the hot stage; and finally the sweating stage, indicating resolution. The initial morbid impression spread by sympathy to weaken the energy of the brain and disturb the equilibrium of the circulation.

Using a vigorous metaphor, he compared the vascular reaction in fever to a civil war between the heart and the capillaries. If the circulatory equilibrium was somehow disturbed, the capillaries, by their contraction, threw blood toward the center. Then the heart, in its turn, "labors, at first in vain, to project it back again" (ibid., pp. 27–30). For recovery, the heart must gain victory over the capillaries and convert the "general *centripetal* into general *centrifugal* action" (p. 35). Only when the equilibrium was reestablished could there be a cure.

For him as for Broussais, disturbance of gastric function was an important clinical feature of fevers. When gastric function was deranged, its sympathies became "deleterious to other parts." The stomach was thus "a centre of sympathetic governance" (pp. 43–44). *Sympathy* he defined as that property whereby *"impression* or *action* in one part, produces impression or action in another" (p. 60).

Caldwell paid relatively little attention to inflammation as a process but kept referring to it as "local affection." It was thus only a severe form of congestion. A simple congestion would be resolved "by a mere increase of excitement," that is, increased action of the heart alone. A more intense grade, however "is too deep to be resolved by reaction short of inflammatory."

Like Broussais and Clutterbuck, Caldwell denied the existence of essential or idiopathic fevers. All fevers, he declared, had a local origin, where the causative agent first made contact and exerted its action. Many different conditions could cause fevers: infection, contagion, cold, atmospheric changes, humidity, unwholesome food or drink, poisonous substances, and passions of the mind. These would be among the so-called remote causes of fever.

Despite their variety, all these factors, he insisted, would affect the body only where actual contact took place. This contact, or "primary impression," could occur in only four areas, namely, the skin, the mucosa of the gastrointestinal tract, the mucosa of the respiratory system, and the brain (where the "passions of the mind" made their first impression directly on the nerve tissue).

He denied that any fever-producing agent had to enter the blood as the first and preliminary step in exerting its action. He denied, furthermore, that an injurious agent could traverse the solid tissue (on its way to the blood) without first doing some injury.

This claim he established through logic alone. Anything that entered the blood would necessarily suffer dilution. It was absurd to think that harmful agents could "produce a greater mischief, after they have been weakened by a mixture with the blood," than in the undiluted state. This absurdity "proved" that injurious agents must first act on the solids, and that agents cannot affect the fluids without first affecting the solids (pp. 56–57).

In this way Caldwell utterly rejected any notion of a *contagium vivum* or of a "ferment" exerting action on the blood. Such explanation offered for fevers had been arousing interest among progressive scientists. Indeed, Caldwell became a bitter opponent of Justus von Liebig and "animal chemistry" and remained a staunch supporter of the solidism that Cullen had popularized.[32] Caldwell rejected the new humoralism that by that time was already making fruitful progress and would soon exert even greater influence.

Caldwell explained fever in purely local terms. Any causative agents first make a "local impression." This "original deleterious impression" generates a "morbid irritation," which in turn "debilitates" the vessels. Because of this, the capillaries cannot act with sufficient vigor to "force the blood onwards . . . as rapidly as it is thrown into them." Hence the blood necessarily accumulates, and the fever "arises *immediately* from *congestion*." He asserted, aggressively, "if there be any thing certain in pathology, it is that fever arises from a primary local affection . . . it is always a *general derangement* proceeding from a *local* cause."[33]

Caldwell's presentations of theory reveal his priorities. Despite all his incursions into theory, his important concern was not the conceptual aspects but the practical implications of the diagnosis. When he felt the pulse, "a quickness or short jerk in the beat. . . . testifies to the existence of topical inflammation" (ibid., p. 49). He diagnosed inflammation from tenuous physical signs. And when he had made the diagnosis, he knew what to do—bleed the patient. He was interested in practice, not in explanation.

Caldwell never emerged from the limitations of the eighteenth century. He did not seek new empirical knowledge or any additional evidence for older concepts. Even though he was constantly asserting his own originality and independence, he depended on the data enunciated by others but enhanced by slippery reasoning. He "solved" the problems of pathogenesis by elaborating theories characteristic of the eighteenth century.

Although Caldwell and Broussais both failed to enter the mainstream of nineteenth-century medicine, a considerable gulf separates them and distinguishes their teachings. Broussais, despite his grave deficiencies, was indeed touched by the new investigative spirit, and he did make extensive autopsy studies. However, he severely misinterpreted his data and he conspicuously lacked a critical spirit. Even though he tried, he could not transcend the stifling passion that characterized so much eighteenth-century thinking—the drive to create systems. Still, he had emerged into the nineteenth-century thought modes, and his stumbling efforts did stimulate younger men to absorb what was new and good. Caldwell, on the other hand, directed his students to ignore the new and persist in the old modes, untouched by progress.

4

The Search for Specificity

THE NINETEENTH-CENTURY PHYSICIANS STRUGGLED with a legacy of problems, of which the nature of fevers was perhaps the most difficult. Cullen, as we have seen, offered his own influential analysis and a classification that served as a foundation for later work. Physicians who followed him in the early nineteenth century acquired only a modest amount of new information. While they sometimes seemed to realize that their knowledge was incomplete, they nevertheless continued to devise explanations from the available concepts. Eventually, new data led to new theories and then to new explanations.

Especially troublesome were the so-called primary fevers, which were of two main types—intermittent fevers, of which our malaria offered a paradigm; and continued fevers, which had an uninterrupted course. In this latter group, Cullen identified three subgroups, the synocha, in which the patient showed a vigorous bodily reaction with a strong pulse and which corresponded to the inflammatory fever of earlier authors; typhus, which showed prostration, feeble pulse, and clouded consciousness; and synochus, which started as the inflammatory synocha but turned into the typhus form. In this chapter I will analyze the way that physicians tried to clarify the concept of typhus and the progress made toward the concept of specificity, in the nineteenth-century sense.

The designation typhus lacked precision, and the diagnosis depended on a few characteristics making up an indefinite pattern.

Cullen defined the pattern in these words: "A contagious disease, body heat only moderately increased, pulse weak, for the most part rapid, sensory functions very much disturbed, severe prostration."[1]

This definition would apply to a wide spectrum of cases. Then the question arose whether the pattern marked out a discrete or specific disease, and whether every case that showed these features represented the same disease. In trying to reach an answer, physicians had as a model the disease smallpox. This was known to Galen, had been clearly described in the tenth century, and exhibited a remarkable uniformity from then to the present. Whatever a disease entity might be, smallpox most assuredly was an instance.

To what extent was typhus (as Cullen conceived it) a disease entity in the same sense? The answer might depend on the degree to which Cullen's typhus resembled smallpox. A fruitful approach to this difficult question lies through the notion of a specific disease.

THE MEANING OF SPECIFIC

The term *specific* is used in two somewhat divergent senses, one approximate and popular, the other precise through its dependence on formal logic. The popular usage refers to something readily identifiable and not likely to be confused with anything else. Without any formal definition or reasoned circumscription, there is a sort of intuitive identification, a recognition stemming from experience and preceding any rational analysis.

Small children, getting acquainted with the world, will quickly learn to distinguish a dog from a cat, and soon will realize that a poodle and a terrier, although quite different, are both "dog." If, after they achieved a certain amount of discrimination, they go to the zoo and see a coyote, a dingo, a wolf, and a fox, they may be puzzled. They might point to these animals and ask, with an inquiring lilt, "Dog?" Their parents might provide an answer based on intuition but not on science.

Science would provide answers based on rational discrimination, on the concept of genera and species and the apparatus of formal classification. Here we encounter the other and more precise meaning of *specific*, namely, the characteristics that demarcate a species—specificity in the strict sense.

Classification—literally, the making of classes—is the process by which individuals, whether postage stamps, animals, or diseases, are arranged into groups showing certain resemblances. These groups, in turn, are arranged according to their degree of inclusiveness. A more inclusive class is called a *genus*, the less inclusive, a *species*, and from these nouns we derive the adjectives *general* and *specific*. If a species can be further subdivided, it becomes a genus, harboring subordinate species. A whole hierarchy of subdivisions can be established, each stage of which may bear a separate name, such as phylum, class, order, or family, and many many more. These refer to degree of inclusiveness. They do not affect the basic relationship of a more inclusive group, whose properties are general, and a subordinate group, more limited, with properties that are more specific.

When pathologists made a formal classification for diseases, known as nosology, they created a hierarchical arrangement exhibiting the basic relation of the more inclusive and the less inclusive, the more general and the more specific. I will restrict myself to the terms *genus* and *species* and avoid any confusing reference to other designations in the hierarchy of division.

Smallpox was the prime example of a specific disease. It is part of a larger group called the exanthemata, which includes measles and chickenpox and whose members all have certain features in common. Exanthems are infectious, they affect a person only once in a lifetime, they produce lesions on the skin, and they have certain similarities in their clinical course. At the same time, they have identifiable differences that permit distinction of one from another. The features they have in common characterize the genus, or superordinate class; the features unique to each identify the species, or subordinate class. Smallpox is a species that can be precisely identified through its own characteristics, often called peculiar or particular. Because they are species, each of the exanthemata is properly called specific.

In symbolic terms we may represent the genus by the letter A and the species by subclasses A' and A''. All the members have certain identities, namely A, and also certain unique differences, expressed by the prime marks. Smallpox would be A', chicken pox, A''. Then the question remains whether this neat formulation, logically impeccable, applies in fact to diseases as they are encountered.

In the class of exanthemata for which Cullen had provided a

definition, he also included the diseases scarlet fever and urticaria (among others). He thought they were distinct species of the exanthems, $(A'''$ and $A'''')$. Today we deny that these belong to the exanthems. Even though they both affect the skin, they diverge in other respects from the asserted definition. In symbolic terms, Cullen would have said that diseases C' and F' belonged in the category A and were thus cognate to A' and A''.

Scarlet fever is certainly a clearly recognizable disease and therefore specific in the popular sense. But in logic it is not a species within its asserted genus. We see the error; Cullen did not. New evidence and new ways of thinking were needed to change the viewpoint.

THE TYPHUS PROBLEM

We can apply these examples to the problem of typhus. In the eighteenth century, a great number of epidemics were described under various names. In Cullen's nosology, when he identified typhus he gave several pages to enumerating such reports under various names. Regardless of the multiplicity of names, he thought he was dealing with a single disease. He referred to the various names not even as varieties of typhus but as synonyms (ibid., pp. 254–57).

We now know that he was dealing with two entirely distinct diseases. One, which we still call typhus, is a louse-borne infection induced by a particular group of microorganisms called rickettsia. The other disease, now identified as typhoid fever, is induced by a particular bacillus, now called salmonella. The mixture of the two diseases led to confusion, whose resolution provides insight into the thought processes of the era. The separation of the two types took place in the 1830s and 1840s, and will be discussed in chapter 5.

During and after the Napoleonic wars there were severe epidemics of rickettsial typhus, a disease even then known to be associated with overcrowding and poverty. One epidemic, which spread to the United States, was responsible for the death of Benjamin Rush, in 1813. The rickettsial typhus did not for many years pose any further major problem in the United States, although epidemics continued to attack Europe. The rickettsial form, true typhus, was quite prevalent in Great Britain, especially in Ireland.

In France, the bacillary type—our typhoid fever—was more prevalent. Physicians in both countries, however, kept referring to a single disease.

Even though Cullen lumped the two forms together as a single specific entity with a single name, he nevertheless seemed troubled by vague doubts. It was possible, he said, that typhus itself was a genus that included several species not as yet identified, but he refused to commit himself. The observations did not necessarily imply specific differences but might be merely varieties, "arising from a different degree of power in the cause," or from different attendant circumstances.[2]

Here we have a profound problem, which Cullen recognized but could not solve. How does a species differ from a variety? A species has certain essential and constant features that define it. Once these have been determined, other features, which may or may not be present, will not affect the specificity. A petunia may be blue or red and a dog may have long hair or short hair, but these features are not relevant to their respective identity as species. Inconstant features, whose presence or absence do not affect the identity as species, were in logic called accidents.

All members of a species have the same unique essence. In a variety, essential characters remain constant, and differences affect only features of secondary importance. In the nineteenth century, when physicians noted the differences between the two forms of typhus, they disputed whether one was a variety of the other, or whether there were two separate species. Any such dispute tells us that the essence of the disease, whatever it might be, had not as yet been determined, at least to general satisfaction.

In framing a definition that identifies a species and discriminates it from all others, the great problem is to determine just which observed properties are in fact essential. The central problem in pathology might be phrased as the search for essence. Any such determination depends not on logic but on empirical observations, critically examined. Cullen did not explicitly phrase the problem in this fashion, but I believe he at least glimpsed it in a hazy fashion.

CONTAGION

Another concept, important in the growth of medical thought, was contagion, already touched on in the preceding chapter. A disease such as smallpox was called contagious if it could spread from one person to another through contact. This term *contagion* referred not only to the process of spread but to the active agent that transmitted the disease. It was a material entity that could act directly, through person-to-person contact, or indirectly, through intermediate substances called fomites. Examples of fomites are cloth, or leather, or other inert material that could carry the pathogenic agent from the affected person to someone else, far removed from the original source.

A great deal of attention was paid to the specificity of a contagion. Smallpox offered the prime example. Cullen considered this to be "a disease arising from a contagion of a specific nature, which produces a fever" and all the rest of the symptoms (see ibid., par. 587). In the early nineteenth century, this concept of specificity was greatly elaborated, but even for Cullen it seemed to mean that the disease could not occur without the presence of that agent.

Cullen recognized two types of smallpox, the discrete and the confluent, of which the latter was the more severe. He queried whether these clinical differences might depend "upon a difference of the contagion producing the disease," but he rejected this supposition. More likely, he thought, the factors responsible for the clinical differences depended not on the contagion itself but on "the state of the person in whom it is applied" or other such circumstance (par. 595).

In a specific contagious disease, Cullen thus recognized two factors. One was the actual contagion, which induced the disease, the other the "circumstances" operative at the time, whether internally, within the individual, or externally, in the environment. Both of these factors, according to the terminology of the time, were remote causes. In the first half of the nineteenth century, the different kinds of remote causes and the concept of specificity were greatly elaborated. Cullen had laid the groundwork for discussion.

MIASMA

In contrast to a contagion, which spread a disease by contact, whether direct or indirect, was a miasma, deemed responsible for certain diseases that did not spread by contact. The prime example here was the intermittent fevers, our malaria. This type of fever did not spread by contact, even of the most intimate kind. It was not "catching." Healthy persons could, with impunity, take care of the sick, with no fear of getting the disease.

Miasma was an exhalation occurring in warm regions and arising from swamps and marshes. It could remain in the atmosphere and induce intermittent fever in those exposed to it. Considerable indirect knowledge accumulated regarding its properties, which I will consider later.

Contagion and miasma produced disease of different types. Cullen attempted a generalization, applicable to both contagions and miasmata, namely, that "some matter floating in the atmosphere, and applied to the bodies of men, ought to be considered the remote cause of fevers" (par. 78). A contagion could enter the atmosphere. A miasma was already there. He believed "that the remote causes of fevers are chiefly Contagions or Miasmata, and neither of them of great variety . . . [and] it will be proper to distinguish the causes of fevers, by using the terms *Human* or *Marsh Effluvia,* rather than the general ones of Contagion or Miasma" (par. 85). A human effluvium was a contagion proceeding from a human body; a marsh effluvium, on the other hand, arose from decaying vegetable matter. This notion of effluvium proved to be a fruitful concept in the early nineteenth century, when the doctrines of Cullen were attacked and modified.

The concept of specificity suggested particular relationships, admittedly obscure, between the "causes" of the disease and the observed clinical phenomena. Cullen laid a framework for later developments that would lead eventually to germ theory and the specificity thereby achieved.

CLASSIFYING BY CAUSE: JOHN ARMSTRONG

During the early nineteenth century, Cullen's views became extensively modified, a process with which John Armstrong (1784–1829) had much to do. He did not uncover any new facts or investigate new data, but he did offer a different way of looking at things.

Armstrong was trained in Edinburgh, where he received the M.D. degree in 1807. In 1816, after major epidemics of typhus had swept over Europe and the United States, he wrote a highly successful book on that disease. The work had three editions in three years, and in 1821 the third British edition was reprinted in

Philadelphia. A second American edition, the next year, suggests the influence he exerted in this country.[3]

Armstrong rejected the current nosologies, which rested on the principle that symptoms would reveal the essence of disease and provide the constant and specific features through which it could be identified. He denied that the clinical characteristics could furnish the proper base for classifying fevers. Analysis by causes, he felt, would offer a much sounder method.

This emphasis on cause as the basis for classifying disease seems to have a fine modern sound, but the appearance is rather deceptive. Armstrong, for the most part quite uncritical, actually introduced much confusion. But he did emphasize a different approach: in his own rather muddy fashion he called attention to some important problems of specificity and their relation to causes.

An emphasis on causation was nothing new. Early in the eighteenth century, Boerhaave, in analyzing disease, had stressed causal factors. His analysis, however, rested not on direct empirical data but on hypothetical entities, acting in a hypothetical fashion. Some ailments, for example, he attributed to an excessive stiffness (or else excessive laxity) of the elemental fibers, but neither the fibers themselves nor any changes in their stiffness had been empirically demonstrated. Similarly, with such alleged causes as an acid or alkaline acrimony, hypothetical agents were derived by analogy. Classical nosology, spearheaded by Boissier de Sauvages, had rejected such hypothetical causes in favor of the directly observed symptoms.[4]

By the late eighteenth century, a great deal of new empirical data on fevers had accumulated, derived largely from study of epidemics. When Armstrong classified fevers, he went back to the notion of cause, but not in a speculative sense. Instead, he relied on concrete observation. He rejected Cullen's claim that synocha, a noncontagious disease, could change into typhus, which was contagious. If one disease could change into another, the notion of specificity was destroyed.

This difficulty Armstrong tried to eliminate through a new grouping. He maintained the basic principle that certain fevers had specific causes that rendered them unique and unchangeable. Other fevers, however, which had general causes, might undergo changes in character. Of the specific fevers he distinguished two types. One was contagious and was transmitted by a contagion. The other, not capable of direct transmission, was noncontagious. Here the responsible agent was a miasma, exerting its effect from the atmosphere. These two agents, each of them specific, could not change into one another.

There remained a class of fevers whose causes were not specific, but general. This whole group he designated as common continued fever, resulting from such "general" causes as cold or heat, or passions of the mind, or other indefinite factors. A specific cause could produce only one kind of disease; a general cause, on the other hand, could produce quite varied diseases, none of them specific.

This analysis provided a nominal classification, intended to bring order into the confusing array of fevers. Armstrong divided all the febrile diseases into two groups, one of which resulted from specific causes, the other from general causes. Fevers with a specific cause he further divided into two types. One, the contagious typhus, was induced by a specific contagion. Correlatively, in the noncontagious type, the specific agent was a miasma.[5]

TYPHUS AS A SPECIFIC CONTAGION

The term *typhus* Armstrong limited to "the peculiar disease" that originates "from a specific contagion" and which can "produce an affection of its own nature" in those exposed to its influence. Nevertheless, typhus "admits to a subordinate division" (ibid., p. 14). Some forms affect the same individual only once, while others can attack repeatedly. All of them, however, have the common characteristic of "arising from, and propagating themselves by peculiar contagions." He regarded typhus as an aggregate of varieties (p. 14). While these had clinical differences, they all showed the same defining feature: origin from a specific contagion. The specificity lay in the alleged cause, not in clinical manifestations.

Here we see the problem of distinguishing between a species and a variety. What Armstrong called typhus and regarded as specific was a whole group of conditions. Typhus, he said, had three different clinical forms, which he called varieties. These, apparently, might pass on into another, without sharp differentiation (p. 19). It did not seem important whether the symptoms were constant, so long as the cause was the same. It is not clear, however, whether the contagion was single or multiple. He used the term sometimes in the singular, sometimes in the plural, but he did not provide any characterization. For Armstrong *contagion* represented little more than a word for the contagious property found in a group of conditions.

The varieties of typhus Armstrong characterized by the physiological processes that were taking place in the body. The first variety was simple typhus, in which an excitement of the heart and vessels (i.e., the febrile reaction) affected the whole system but without giving any signs of local inflammation. There was a uniform distribution of blood through the system. Any minor congestions might be dissipated "by the energies of the constitution alone" or by very mild medication (p. 25). This form had a fairly straightforward clinical course. In fatal cases, autopsy showed very little anatomic change, but he suspected that there might be undiscovered lesions, "perhaps many morbid changes, which elude the inquisition of the anatomist." Without more knowledge, he said, we cannot expect to find any "slender and latent lesions" (p. 23).

A second variety of typhus showed a different form of pathogenesis. If the blood became "superabundant in particular parts," inflammation supervened, and the local accumulation would no longer yield to simple action of the circulatory system. This feature characterized inflammatory typhus, which might affect three main regions—the brain, the lungs, and the abdominal organs. Symptoms, obviously, would vary according to the character of the inflammation and the part affected, but in all, "the genuine marks of inflammation mark it as one affection" (p. 38). Anyone ignorant of "modern pathology," he said, would be very surprised to learn that a patient with inflammation of the brain, another with inflammation of the lungs, and a third with inflammation of the bowel were all suffering from the same disease. Yet, he went on, "this would be as legitimate a generalization as any in physic" (p. 60).

The third variety, congestive typhus, showed an absence of excitement. Inflammatory typhus resulted from an increased action of the heart (i.e., excitement). Symmetry called for the opposite type of pathogenesis, with diminished action of the heart. This fascinating category, widely recognized, we will discuss in detail in chapter 6.

Through his classification, I suggest, Armstrong wanted to establish a principle that contradicted Cullen: a contagious disease cannot arise from one that is not contagious. If we wanted to know why, he would answer that the causes were different, and the cause determines the disease. This insight is Armstrong's real contribution.

The different forms of typhus might be difficult to separate clinically, but they were all subsumed under a single name that indicated a common property, namely, that all were caused by contagion. After presenting this major principle, Armstrong discussed clinical symptoms and indications for treatment. He gave many individual case histories, with different clinical findings. The cases were all assumed, without proof, to be one or another form of typhus. While he called them all the same disease, he was actually begging the question and assuming what had to be proved. Moreover, in his discussion of individual cases of typhus, there was no evidence that they involved contagion.

I give an example of what he called inflammatory typhus, of the cerebral form. He described "an old and corpulent lady laboring under typhus," in whom there was "an excessive disturbance in the circulation of the head, and an almost incessant sickness of the stomach." The cephalic symptoms increased. On the fourth day she had a hemiplegia with blindness in one eye. Although she had been affected "with great intellectual disorder," she became quite clear, mentally, for several hours. Then she gradually lapsed into a coma and expired in convulsions. This, he thought, represented typhus with inflammation of the brain (pp. 34–35). The modern reader might regard this so-called inflammatory typhus as, perhaps, hypertensive encephalopathy, with cerebral hemorrhage.

The specificity of diseases such as smallpox or intermittent fever involved two components, observable clinical patterns and the actual responsible agents—the contagion and the miasma, respectively. Clinical patterns were sharply defined and would not be confused with other clinical conditions. For comparison with typhus, as Armstrong conceived it, we might review some data about the responsible agents.

The contagion of smallpox had not been isolated and empirically demonstrated—that would come only in the twentieth century—but some of its properties were known. I would mention, for example, the variation in virulence, the ability to induce immunity, the relationship to cowpox, and the abundant evidence on the various modes of transmission. This was a substantial quantity of knowledge, derived from the study of the effects. The agent, however, was still a hypothetical entity, a construct elaborated from observation of its effects.

Pathologists reasoned backward from the observed effects to the properties of the cause. These various aspects of the disease, which revealed the properties of the cause, were regular, predictable, and clearly recognizable. The contagion of smallpox was accepted as specific because the clinical disease was sharply defined. The specificity of the agent depended on the specificity of the disease it was supposed to induce.

Similarly with the noncontagious miasma, the agent of intermittent fever. Despite many attempts, it had never been isolated, yet its effects—the disease—correlated strongly with certain details known about the agent. Thus, the disease was associated with marshy land, stagnant water, and a warm climate, yet the agent could not pass over large bodies of water. There was special activity in the early morning and the evening. Winds could carry miasma long distances, but altitude offered a protection. Knowledge concerning such properties of miasma were greatly elaborated later in the century.[6] These enumerated properties, we now know, actually refer to the mosquito, which, however, still comprises a "remote cause" of clinical malaria.

If, now, we regard the alleged specificity of typhus (as Armstrong defined it), we find a vastly different situation. When we speak of a specific cause, whether proximal or remote, we must keep in mind the question, Cause of what? Instead of giving us a circumscribed clinical pattern, clearly recognizable as an effect of the alleged cause, Armstrong lumped together as the effect a wide range of disparate clinical patterns. Unity was conferred only by the name. Then, to the entire aggregate of clinical findings, he assigned an allegedly specific cause. But if the effects lacked constancy, how could the properties of the alleged cause be identified or its nature inferred? Attribution of a specific cause to Armstrong's typhus lacked the cogency that attended a comparable assertion about smallpox.

Armstrong's claim of a specific cause for typhus failed completely, because we do not know what it was the cause *of*, that is, what constant effect the supposedly specific cause produced. We have a wonderful circularity. The disease was considered specific because it had specific cause. The cause was specific because it produced specific disease.

With the wisdom of retrospection we note Armstrong's positive contribution. He recognized that typhus, as then understood, was highly complex, and for its elucidation a reliance on clinical symptoms was not good enough. A new approach, through the study of causes, was preferable, but he did not know how to proceed. He had no notion of systematic investigation or effective demonstration. Yet in pursuing his views, he maintained that the nature of the cause determined the nature of the fever, and one fever could not change into another. He also wanted to break away from the confines of Cullen's system and to refute the concept of synochus. His earlier work marked a real, even if somewhat hazy, advance toward modern views.

ARMSTRONG'S CHANGE OF MIND

One of the great ironies of medical history is the way that Armstrong, before his death, completely changed his mind regarding the specificity of disease. He described the change in a posthumously published text. In the 1820s Armstrong had given lectures, which a student had transcribed. Before he died, Armstrong saw this transcript and, in a letter, attested to its accuracy. The transcription, together with the letter of attestation, was published in England in 1834. In 1837 an American edition appeared in Philadelphia.[7]

The text, somewhat cursory, showed a radical change of mind, described with great humility. In typhus he admitted having "strenuously maintained the doctrine of human contagion." But then, he declared, he "met with a case of intermittent fever. In a few days the fever became remittent, and in a few days more it put on the continued character, and the patient died with all the most malignant symptoms of typhus fever" (ibid., vol. 2, p. 113). We do not know how many cases of this character he encountered.

Contrary to what he had claimed earlier, Armstrong now believed that typhus resulted not from a specific contagion but from an "exhalation connected with certain states of the earth and air" (i.e., miasma). He declared, "I am perfectly convinced that what is commonly called typhus fever does arise from malaria, or marsh effluvia; that it is intermittent, remittent, and continued; . . . and that it does not originate from human contagion." This case (presumably an example of aestivo-autumnal malaria, to be discussed later) related to the so-called typhomalaria.[8]

In his posthumous book, Armstrong thus regarded typhus as a miasmatic rather than a contagious disease. He became convinced that miasma "produces an intermittent, a remittent, and a continued form of fever; each form having a peculiar set of symptoms, and each passing and repassing into the other forms, so as to completely identify them as mere variations of one and the same disease."[9] As I interpret his discussion, typhus had lost all status of specificity and had become a typhoid state, such as Benjamin Rush had discussed, rather than a disease, sui generis.

Armstrong failed to pierce the obscurity surrounding the different kinds of fever, for he lacked the methodology, techniques, and concepts that French and German investigators were slowly forging at that time. The path of eventual clarity would lie through regions of "animal chemistry," cell theory, and physiology. These, however, along with new modes of thinking, were fields that Armstrong could not enter. In the next half a century or so, the emerging science of bacteriology would throw light on problems that troubled him but would in turn introduce new problems to puzzle his successors.

NATHAN SMITH'S CIRCUMSCRIPTION OF "TYPHOUS FEVER"

If we pass from the highly trained physicians of Edinburgh or London to a poorly trained rural practitioner of New England, we get a different appreciation of medical progress. We see that medical sophistication holds less importance than does the insight, discrimination, and critical judgment of the investigator.

In the nineteenth century, many prominent American physicians, showing these qualities to a high degree, came from a humble background, with only a meager formal education. Such a one was Nathan Smith (1762–1829), who was born in a small farming community in Massachusetts. His father soon migrated to Chester, Vermont, then an unsettled area, where the boy had but a desultory education. The story is told that when Smith was twenty-one years old, a surgeon came to his community to perform an amputation. Smith assisted in the operation, an experience that kindled his desire to study medicine. After a year spent in improving his general education, Smith was apprenticed to that same surgeon for the customary three-year period. This training qualified him to practice, and in 1787 he settled in New Hampshire, about twenty miles from Hanover.

Soon realizing the deficiencies in his training, Smith determined to attend medical school. The nearest was the Harvard Medical School in Boston, established in 1783. The course of lectures were short and the clinical instruction scanty. For three years Smith attended lectures, and in 1790 he received the degree of Bachelor of Medicine.

Then Smith conceived the idea of starting a new medical school in New Hampshire. In 1796 he applied to the trustees of Dartmouth College for sponsorship. Not discouraged by the rather equivocal response, he went abroad for six months, attending lectures and hospital practice in both Edinburgh and London and collecting books and apparatus for the new school.

The medical school at Dartmouth, with Smith as virtually a one-man faculty, was officially established in 1798. By 1812, sixty-four medical students had received the degree of Bachelor of Medicine, with Smith furnishing most of the instruction. In 1812 he accepted a call from the newly founded medical school at Yale, in New Haven, and continued teaching there until his death in 1829.[10] Smith achieved an important niche in the history of education, but for our purpose his study of typhus was more important.

In the sparsely settled United States, *typhus* was a popular diagnostic term, but it lacked any clear meaning. In Philadelphia in 1834 statistics regarding the causes of death provided a category of fever, and then enumerated eleven different kinds: typhus, scarlet, bilious, catarrhal, remittent, intermittent, puerperal, eruptive, hectic, continued, and putrid. Diseases like smallpox and measles had separate individual listings.[11] Even though there was considerable discrimination, diagnostic criteria were not precise. The list was not exhaustive, and still further diagnoses would be readily made, especially in smaller communities.

From his many years of observation, Smith had a distinct insight that certain cases described under various names, such as long fever, slow fever, nervous fever, and putrid fever, formed a distinct pattern, which could be discriminated from all others. In 1824 he published his monograph, *Practical Essay on Typhous Fever*, which, though not much appreciated in his own time, is one of the classics of American medicine.[12]

Typhous, of course, is the proper adjectival form of the noun *typhus*, more precise than *typhoid*, which merely denotes something typhuslike. At the time that Smith wrote, a distinction between typhous and typhoid might seem trivial. Only in the next decade did the distinction become important.

Typhoid fever, the disease Smith studied under the diagnosis of typhus, was endemic in the United States. He regarded it as a specific disease, sui generis, with its own "characteristic marks." It occurred in all parts of the United States and in every month of the year. Smith's many years of practice led him to say, "I consider Typhous Fever a disease *sui generis,* arising from a specific cause, and that cause contagion, and seldom affecting the same person more than once" (ibid., pp. 788–89).

However, if it was really a disease in its own right, with its own unique character, not to be confused with any other, how could it be circumscribed and identified? Armstrong, when discussing typhus, did not even try to make any precise separations. Smith, using the same diagnostic term, devoted himself to making a distinction as precise as possible. He was referring to bacillary typhus, which in Great Britain was not discriminated from the more common rickettsial typhus.

The eventual separation, we will discuss in the next chapter; here I am concerned with Smith's methods of investigation and his views on specificity and contagion. In asserting a clearly defined entity, he relied principally on analogy, an indirect mode of investigation. Having accumulated abundant observations on febrile diseases, he had the flash of insight of a close similarity that a particular group bore to smallpox. If the latter were sui generis, so too was typhous fever. He perceived a definitive pattern.

Firmly believing in the specificity of the disease, Smith offered his reasons in concise fashion. A key feature was the concept of contagion. Refusing to be drawn into any controversy regarding contagion versus infection, Smith declared, "By a contagious disease, I mean simply, one that can be communicated from one individual to another" (p. 784). The prime example of a contagious disease was smallpox.

Since at least the sixteenth century, physicians realized that contagious diseases could spread by the transfer of imperceptible particles from one person to another, either directly, or else indirectly through fomites. Furthermore, such contact was the only mode of spread. Smallpox, for example, would come only from a previously infected person. It did not arise "spontaneously." Another feature of smallpox, already noted, was the immunity that one attack produced.

Unlike contemporary French investigators, Smith did not collect data systematically. He employed no quantitative methods, he performed no autopsies, and he did not tabulate his data. Instead, he had a sort of "aha!" reaction, by which he perceived a discrete pattern within a multiplicity of data.

Smith asserted that typhous fever was contagious. Some writers denied this on the grounds that in an epidemic not every exposed person contracted the disease. But this, Smith pointed out, was equally true of smallpox, universally accepted as contagious. A further objection declared that the disease might appear where a source (i.e., an infected person responsible for the transmission) could not be identified. Those who offered this objection were denying any specific or unique cause and implying that the disease in question could arise from nonspecific environmental factors, or so-called general causes.

In rebuttal, Smith provided good epidemiological evidence. He pointed to clusters of cases he had traced to persons who had recently arrived from a community where they had come in contact with the same disease. Studying the spread of the disease was not too difficult in the sparsely populated country. A few examples with clear evidence of contagion were far more convincing than a large number of cases where no origin could be traced. Smith declared, somewhat cavalierly, "A few instances, which have fallen under my own observation, would alone be sufficient to determine the question" (p. 784).

Smith rejected the notion of general causes. Some physicians, while admitting the spread of typhous fever, held that it arose not from specific contagion but rather "from errors in diet or exercise, from the effects of temperature, or what Sydenham would call an epidemic state of the atmosphere, from marsh miasmata, or confinement in close and crowded apartments" (p. 785).

This objection Smith rebutted through reasoning. From his own experience he knew that some regions of the country might be free of the disease for as long as twenty years. Could the nonspecific factors, mentioned above, fail to occur at least some time during these long periods? If the disease actually did arise from nonspecific factors, as was claimed, "it is impossible but that some of these circumstances should have occurred" during the time in question (p. 785).

In comparable fashion, Smith discussed the belief that typhous fever might arise from the same marsh miasmata that produced intermittent fever. This, too, he rebutted by logic. In a very large area, more than two hundred miles across, he said, no one had ever contracted intermittent fever, yet typhous fever was widely prevalent there. Thus, using what John Stuart Mill would later call the canons of induction, Smith felt that he could rule out certain alleged causes of typhous fever.

Knowing nothing of bacteria, Smith postulated a specific contagion as the agent responsible for the disease. Its nature was unknown, and so too were the ways by which it "operates upon the system," or the locus where it "makes its first impression," or "just how this first impression produces the ultimate effects" (p. 790). He admitted ignorance on these aspects that we now call pathogenesis. However, if a disease "can be communicated from one person to another, it has a specific cause, and I know no disease that arises from a specific cause, that can be produced without the agency of that cause" (p. 785). Diffuse and nonspecific environmental factors could not induce typhous fever.

Yet Smith was waging an uphill battle. Most physicians in the community regarded various environmental factors as probable causal agents in disease. Smith realized that these popularly accepted factors lacked any logical force. On the other hand, a specific agent that was only postulated but not directly observed, whose very existence could be inferred only from its effects, carried little conviction to most physicians. Furthermore, typhous fever had no pathognomonic or even striking clinical symptoms, but the diagnosis depended rather on a whole pattern. Under such circumstances, accepting the real existence of some undefined specific agent required an act of faith. Smith had that faith, which he justified by theoretical considerations, clinical experience, and analogy, but he could not convince others.

ARGUMENTS FOR SPECIFICITY

An important argument for specificity rested on the immunity that a single attack conferred. If the analogy with smallpox were to hold, a patient who recovered from one attack of typhous fever would not contract it a second time. Smith regarded this as an established fact, and any opposition to this view had its origin, he thought, in faulty diagnosis. Many physicians, he said, gave the name typhus to a wide range of other diseases, such as "catarrhal fever," or perhaps "bilious affections," or a variety of "stomach complaints." If physicians diagnosed typhous fever correctly and kept it distinct from other patterns superficially similar, there would be no doubt that one attack conveyed immunity. If diagnosis was wrong, patients might seem to have contracted typhous fever more than once, when actually they had two quite different diseases. Assertions of immunity depended on correct diagnosis (p. 789).

Unfortunately, there was no agreement on just how this disease could be rigorously identified. Diagnostic criteria were lax, and the terms *low fever* and *nervous fever* were applied to a range of gastrointestinal disturbances. Anyone so unskillful as to "call a stomach affection typhus, would be equally liable to call other febrile complaints by the same name" (p. 787).

Smith admitted the difficulty of diagnosis. In its first stages, the disease "exhibits so many symptoms in common with other febrile affections, that it is not easy for anyone, especially the unexperienced, to determine whether the disease is really Typhous Fever or not." Even experienced physicians could not make a diagnosis "till the disease has, in a considerable degree, developed itself" (p. 800). He was emphasizing the need to consider the whole temporal course of the disease and the pattern it exhibited. As part of his analysis, he described the clinical features. While the acuity of his observations compel admiration, the details do not concern us here.

Specificity of a disease implies an identity throughout its course. Variation in symptoms did not mean that the disease itself had altered. Instead, there was a basic unity that persisted through all the variations. Such a view directly contradicted the theories of Rush, who claimed that one fever could change into another.

If typhus was a specific entity whose progression was determined by its own inner nature, then no treatment administered at the first sign of illness could cut short the disease. In Smith's formulation, "if it [the disease] arises from a specific cause and has a natural termination, it may be a question . . . if we possess the power, [or] whether we can with propriety cut it off in its commencement and by art prevent its running its course?" (p. 799).

The desire to cut short (or, in the idiom of the day, to jugulate) a disease in its early stages had always been widespread. The validity of any such procedure, however, depends partly on the query, Is the diagnosis correct? Does the patient really suffer from the disease in question? Rush, for example, regarded bloodletting as a remedy for fevers once established and also, if performed early, as a means of aborting the disease. When, in 1793, yellow fever invaded Philadelphia, he would bleed patients at the very first sign of illness. His mortality figures were much lower than those of his competitors. For him this proved that bloodletting, if performed early enough, would abort the disease. But how did he know that his patients really had yellow fever? Unless the diagnosis was clearly established, his claims had little force.

Smith believed that while typhous fever was a specific disease, the diagnosis could not be made until characteristic features had become manifest. If, relying on early symptoms, a physician diagnosed and treated the disease, and the patient recovered, no conclusion could be drawn regarding the identity of the disease or effectiveness of the therapy. Smith was convinced that in typhous fever treatment could certainly make the patient more comfortable and prevent complications but would not cut short its course.

In all this, Smith was approaching the concept of the self-limited disease. This idea was formally propounded in 1835 in a lecture by Jacob Bigelow (1787–1879).[13] Suffice to note here that Smith had explicitly described most of the points that Bigelow made several years later. Bigelow did indeed mention Smith's work, but only in passing and without any commendation of the splendid insights that antedated his own.

Clearly, Smith was ahead of his time and found little support for his concepts and but little appreciation. He relied on clinical and epidemiological evidence, without the support of anatomical dissections that the French were popularizing. In the intellectual milieu of his period, his work was not cogent enough to convince skeptics.

Nevertheless, he provided a superb example of the scientific method and the new or enlightened empiricism. He collected new observational data, examined them critically, and achieved new but limited conclusions that remained close to the observations. He was not concerned with theorizing that outran the evidence. Compared with the procedures of Louis and other French investigators described in the next chapter, Smith had only scanty evidence for his assertions. He did, however, have clear perception. He firmly demonstrated that the new empiricism demanded a harmonious blend of observation and reasoning, of data and inference. His own careful observations and cautious inferences contrast sharply with the uncritical writings of Armstrong.

SIMPLISTIC THINKING GONE ASTRAY: T. SOUTHWOOD SMITH

In the current of medical thought, Thomas Southwood Smith (1788–1861) provided a modest shift in direction. He first studied for the ministry and was prominent in evangelical and Unitarian circles. However, wanting to combine medical practice with preaching, he entered the medical school in Edinburgh in 1812. Soon after receiving his M.D. degree in 1816, he settled in London. In 1824 he was appointed physician to the London Fever Hospital. Later he became a leader in what was soon called social medicine, with special reference to social betterment, sanitary reform, and public health measures.[14]

For our purposes, the whole sanitary movement has less relevance than Southwood Smith's special analysis of fever. His important book, *A Treatise on Fever*, was published in London in 1830 and immediately reprinted in Philadelphia.[15] His long experience in the Fever Hospital gave his pronouncements special significance for his contemporaries.

Southwood Smith was part of the medical generation still dominated by William Cullen but that nevertheless showed a distinct breaking away in the early nineteenth century. Southwood Smith, trying to clarify the traditional views, depended on both clinical observation and autopsy studies. His analysis took place in the shadow of the older nosology, which by this time was definitely crumbling.

Fever for him was a single genus consisting of several species, each of which presented several varieties. No single characteristic feature identified the "disease." Instead, he said, "fever is a series of events" and research must discover what these events are "and in what order they constantly succeed each other" (ibid., pp. 46–47).

The important aspects of fever did not consist of symptoms, since these, he pointed out, depended on the state of the organs. It was essential to study, rather, the organs themselves. These invariably exhibited certain changes after fever, "from the most trivial intermittent to the most alarming continued fever, from the mildest plague to the most malignant typhus." Fever always affected certain organs, whose identity he inferred from their "disordered function" and the morbid appearances they showed after death. Clinical manifestations allowed him to infer the organs involved, while the morbid appearances found after death provided further evidence (p. 48).

Southwood Smith's analysis shows the influence of Cullen. The organs affected in fever, he declared, are the nervous system, the circulatory system, and the systems of secretion and excretion. For fever to occur, derangement in these organs must take place in a single invariable order. First is involvement of the nervous and sensorial functions, then derangement of the circulatory functions, and finally a disturbance of the secretory and excretory functions. In inflammation (as separate from fever) the same phenomena occur but in a different order (pp. 50–51). His concept of invariable order indicated the importance of pattern, however poorly articulated. While inflammation and fever both showed disturbances in the same organ systems, the disturbances were not the same, since they took place in a different sequence.

To explain the diversity in fever, Southwood Smith introduced a quantitative factor. Some organs were affected to a greater degree than others, and this variation in intensity accounted for the differences in fevers. In one type, perhaps, the nervous system might be most intensely affected, in another, the digestive system. The most severe symptoms would attack one particular component of the "circle" (i.e., the three involved organ systems), while all other organs in the circle would be definitely but less intensely involved.

He gave an example very similar to Armstrong's case noted above. In typhus, he said, the brain may be violently affected and the patient "struck with paralysis or apoplexy," while the digestions and secretions were less severely involved (p. 55). Yet all the organs would be in a morbid state. Even in the intense cerebral affection, which he had no hesitation in diagnosing as typhus, there would always be deranged function in the heart and arteries and in the organs of secretion and excretion.

In no two cases of fever "are all these organs affected in the same degree" (p. 51). Symptoms that reflected altered action depended on organs whose state was constantly varying. Hence, "from one and the same affection, differing only in the degree of its intensity, the symptoms may not only vary but be directly opposite" (p. 59).

In direct contrast, febrile states resulting from a localized inflammation (i.e., the *phlegmasiae*) were not fevers in the strict sense, since they resulted from a different series of phenomena. "There are no fevers but idiopathic fevers" (p. 61), a direct contradiction of Clutterbuck and Broussais. In his discussions of morbid anatomy, this dictum helped to determine which changes should receive attention at post-mortem examination.

While various diseases might be differentiated and named, such a classification really diverts the mind "from dwelling on those essential circumstances which make all of them mere varieties of one great disease" (p. 64–65). The nosologic terms—genera, species, and varieties—only pointed out different degrees of the same malady. They led only to "notions so false and pernicious, that I think it right to abandon the use of them altogether" (p. 71).

He continued, "the more we investigate the subject, the more satisfied we shall become that continued fever is one disease and only one, however varied, or even opposite, the aspect it may present." Every case differed in intensity, "and this alone is the cause of the different forms it [the fever] assumes" (p. 71). Southwood Smith was thus only repeating what Benjamin Rush had already said—there is only one fever, which exhibits different states. He had no sense of qualitative specificity among the fevers.

For practical purposes of nomenclature, the assemblage of symptoms can be arranged into two great classes, "the one comprehending the mild and the other the severe form of the disease" (p. 71). The only real symptoms of debility predominated, the fever was called a typhus. When, on the contrary, inflammatory symptoms were most intense, the fever was called a synocha. Both of these conditions Southwood Smith divided into two forms, the *mitior* and the *gravior*, the less severe and the more severe, respectively. This discrimination had practical importance, for the two forms would require different therapy. However, he offered no criteria for discrimination (pp. 72–73).

Southwood Smith condemned the separation of fevers into various subgroups, such as the exanthemata. Scarlet fever, he believed, was sometimes synochoid and sometimes typhoid, and so too was smallpox. This latter had a peculiar eruption, "but it is as much a genuine fever as typhus, and ought no more to be taken out of this class on account of the eruption upon the skin, than scarlatina." He was thus rejecting Cullen's distinction between the exanthemata and *febres*, or essential fevers. Instead, he categorized the continued fevers into those with and those without eruption and then offered further division into synochoid or typhoid (p. 74).

While Southwood Smith adopted the concepts of Benjamin Rush and to a lesser extent those of John Brown, he differed from them in emphasizing the study of organs through postmortem examination. Symptoms merely expressed an underlying change in the organs, and the important need was to study these changes.

With this in mind, he carried out extensive autopsy studies, which he believed supported his theories. He started out with a fixed idea, that the essential fevers composed a single group, all showing a single pattern of physiological changes. They could be distinguished from the *phlegmasiae*, or fevers that accompanied localized inflammations. The exciting cause of fever was a "poison," whose action depended on quantitative factors. It attacked with variable intensity and affected different organs. In these organs, anatomical changes differed only in intensity of the process. Clinical symptoms, which depended on the particular organs involved, would be proportional to the intensity of the morbid changes (pp. 349–69).

Anatomical studies and clinical observations formed a rigid unit, with each aspect supporting the others. It explained away all apparent exceptions. The whole structure rested on the preexisting idea that essential fever was a unitary entity, with a single cause and a single type of reaction, quite distinct from those febrile reactions that might accompany localized inflammations.

The traditional *phlegmasiae*, which could involve any organ of the body, all had appropriate names, such as pleurisy, arthritis, nephritis, cystitis, and the like. Anatomical changes induced by such disturbances must be kept separate from the alterations associated with the disease entity, essential fever. When Southwood Smith described the morbid changes in fevers, he did not pay attention to whatever changes might be attributed to localized inflammatory diseases.

EVIDENCE MISINTERPRETED

To support his concepts, Southwood Smith presented a great deal of "evidence." Clinically, he had already pointed out that the essential fevers invariably affected first the nervous system, then the cardiovascular system (which included respiratory function), and finally the organs of secretion and excretion. Symptoms like headache or lassitude (Cullen's "debility") were considered to represent nervous system involvement. In a primary inflammation, febrile reactions that might occur never showed nervous system involvement as the first step. In a more modern terminology, he was saying that essential fevers started out with systemic reactions, while the *phlegmasiae* began locally.

When Southwood Smith presented the anatomical changes in fever, he followed a more or less orderly presentation—first the changes in the brian, then in the thorax, and finally in the abdomen. For the brain, he noted that the changes differed greatly from one case to another. He described especially the heightened vascularity and the increase of fluid. The latter would vary in character. It might be clear and serous, or straw colored, or bloody, or opaque and mixed with pus (pp. 182–84). In his more detailed protocols of particular cases, his descriptions suggested such diverse conditions as purulent meningitis, tuberculous meningitis, and "softening," which might represent infarctions. All of these were considered the cerebral pathology in typhus, and this, in turn, was regarded as a single disease, varying only in severity.

For the thorax, he described only the pulmonary changes that could be attributed to essential fevers. He noted but disregarded the primary inflammatory conditions of the lungs, like pneumonia or tuberculosis. He described the congestion and thickening of the bronchial mucosa, deemed constant and characteristic. The substance of the lungs was "engorged with blood or infiltrated with serum," considered to be "essential parts of the morbid phenomena" (p. 186).

Finally, for the abdomen he described in detail the changes in the intestines, already well studied by earlier French pathologists. The lesions, which would soon be recognized as characteristic of typhoid fever, varied in severity, and this feature correlated quite well with the intensity of the clinical phenomena.

Southwood Smith started with the initial bias that, in fever, clinical findings and morbid changes varied only in location and intensity. This, of course, was a massive assumption and a complete *petitio principi*. When, with present knowledge, we study his exposition, we see that the anatomical changes that he described for typhus would also apply to purulent meningitis, cerebral infarction, influenza, and typhoid fever, to mention only the most obvious. According to his assumption, these would be all one disease. In his autopsies he found only what he wanted to find, data to support the claim that the disease differed only in intensity and location.

Since microscopy had as yet no value in analyzing morbid changes, Southwood Smith had to depend on gross appearances. Unlike Giovanni Morgagni, he was not a competent morbid anatomist, and his interpretations were hobbled by his conviction that he dealt with one disease. Believing that clinical and anatomical phenomena in fever varied only quantitatively, he was impervious to qualitatively different patterns. He had attempted a simple reductionism and in so doing revealed all the defects of eighteenth-century thinking to which he had been exposed. But he had not absorbed the new methods that the contemporary French physicians were developing.

Southwood Smith was not an original thinker. His views resembled those of John Armstrong and Henry Clutterbuck and, despite expressed differences, of William Cullen. Each of them claimed that in fever the primary involvement lay in the brain and its special functioning. Armstrong, furthermore, emphasized that various conditions, no matter how different they appeared clinically, were nevertheless only one disease. Qualitative distinctions, although recognized, were considered of no real importance.

The pathologic data, and the inferences that Southwood Smith drew therefrom, were soon rendered obsolete by new advances in microscopy, by anatomy and physiology of the nervous system, and by animal chemistry. When he tried to expound pathology, he showed himself as at the end of an era. A new tide of progress, both conceptual and technological, was bringing new modes of thinking. Southwood Smith would himself contribute to these modes—not, however, in pathology but in the growing movement concerned with public health. This activity forms part of social medicine in its broad sense, but while vastly important in the history of medicine, it lies outside the immediate concern of this book.

A NEW INVESTIGATIVE SPIRIT

Of the physicians we have considered in this chapter, Nathan Smith best represents the progressive movements of the early nineteenth century. Not dependent on theory, he studied a single disease, in which he perceived a clear qualitative pattern that united different types of data. He greatly expanded the "natural history" of the disease. Over the next two decades, more intense study, especially in France and in the United States, would lead to still greater insight.

At the same time, other investigators were pursuing different lines of study. They were concentrating more on the questions of causation and would eventually end up with what is often called the germ theory of disease. The two trends, pursuit of disease patterns and concern with etiology (especially "germs"), would in time merge. But they took different paths and must be considered separately.

5

The Search Partly Successful: The Discrimination of Typhoid Fever

B Y THE BEGINNING OF THE NINETEENTH CENTURY, physicians had described a great many epidemics under such names as jail fever, putrid fever, ship fever, petechial fever, spotted fever, malignant pestilential fever, and many others. However, there was no primary description of any epidemic to which the name *typhus* had been attached. That designation entered the modern literature in the eighteenth century with the development of nosology.

TYPHUS AS A DIAGNOSTIC TERM

The designation *typhus* was the application of an old term in a new sense. It is the English rendition of the Greek word meaning smoke or vapor. By extension, it had taken on the connotation of a clouded sensorium and stupor. As such, it came to indicate certain features prominent in many cases of fever.

That particular sense became useful when physicians realized the importance of classifying diseases in some orderly fashion. In the seventeenth century, we recall, Thomas Sydenham had pleaded for a classification that would eliminate the multiplicity of names that even then proved distressing. With the resulting development of nosology, the name *typhus* usefully identified a particular niche in classification, a niche that would circumscribe certain kinds of fever, regardless of their previous names.

To Boissier de Sauvages, the first modern nosologist, we owe the use of *typhus* to designate a particular disease. He did not employ that term in his early work of 1734, but did use it in 1762. Of the many nosologists who, during the next half century, took turns making new classifications and definitions, some used the term *typhus*, others did not. The designation became generally adopted after William Cullen accepted it in 1772. David Hosack (1769–1835), when he surveyed all the modern nosologies, made it easy for us to note which of the early authors accepted the term and which did not.[1]

The term *typhus* was eventually applied to a wide range of cases described under various names. The original descriptions often permit us, in retrospect, to recognize the original disease. For the most part, these cases fell into the categories we now recognize as either louse-borne typhus ("genuine typhus") or else typhoid fever, of bacterial origin. All of them had gotten lumped together in a single undifferentiated group. The term did not have a sharp denotation. We might speak of "strict constructionists," like Cullen, who limited its application pretty much to the bacterial and rickettsial forms. There were also "loose constructionists," such as Henry Clutterbuck, John Armstrong, and Thomas Southwood Smith, who broadened the extension of typhus to include apoplexy, influenza, and bacterial and other forms of primary meningitis. The different conditions did have in common the manifestations of a clouded mentation and a severe prostration.

The word *typhus* was used in two distinct senses. It could serve as a noun, to designate a febrile disease with certain identifiable properties. Even if these were indefinite and poorly circumscribed, they generally had enough individuality to distinguish the condition from other diseases, such as inflammatory or intermittent fevers.

Benjamin Rush, on the other hand, denied the existence of individual fevers. He regarded typhus as an adjective, that could, for example, describe a typhus state. He also identified a typhoid state (that is, typhuslike, similar but not identical), with a lesser degree of intensity. These states did not have independent stability but could succeed one another, sometimes with considerable rapidity.

In the nineteenth century, it was quite common to read in a case report that a fever "became typhus," meaning that symptoms of stupor and severe debility had occurred. These symptoms could come and go and might attach to any fever. Whenever a fever showed these symptoms, the physician could speak of "a typhus fever."

This adjectival usage did not imply a distinct disease entity (as did the use of *typhus* as a noun) but referred only to certain symptoms observed therein. There was no implication that the original fever had transformed into the particular disease called typhus but only that it assumed some of the symptoms found there. There would have been less confusion if the physician had used the proper adjective *typhoid*, meaning typhuslike, instead of *typhus* in an adjectival sense.

DISEASE AS A PATTERN

When *typhus* was used as a noun, it referred to an entity that was more than merely the loose aggregate of particular symptoms. As a noun, *typhus* meant that the symptoms were not transient phenomena that could come and go in more or less random fashion. Rather, they formed a definite pattern that exhibited a stability and constancy. By pattern, I mean a grouping of features not randomly associated but cohering by virtue of some inner connection.

The essence of a pattern, in this sense, was the coherence and connectedness of its various manifestation and the inner relationship between the individual phenomena. The nature of the connections, or whatever agent was responsible for them, might have been hypothetical, but some agency, known or unknown, provided a connecting link. A pattern was thus a dynamic unity: it exhibited forces that unified the various components.

The discovery or perception of a pattern embodied an act of insight. There was a realization that, of the vast number of observable phenomena, certain ones hung together through an inner connection, while other phenomena were not really relevant. We have seen how Nathan Smith perceived a pattern he called typhous fever, which included not only clinical findings but also epidemiologic and immunologic data. To tie all these phenomena together and to indicate some inner connection binding them into a unity, Smith realized the need of a causal factor. This he could identify only as a contagion. It was postulated, not observed, yet it served to unify and explain the actual observations. Eventually the contagion, which we know as a specific bacterium, was isolated and studied.

The assumption, or postulation, of a causal factor is a recognized mode of scientific research. In the first half of the nineteenth century, perhaps the most brilliant example was the discovery of the planet Neptune. To account for certain irregularities in the orbit of the planet Uranus, the existence of some unknown planet was postulated. Eventually, the hypothetical agent, now known as the planet Neptune, was empirically demonstrated. From the constant observed phenomena, regarded as effects, scientists eventually demonstrated a cause.

In medicine, Smith postulated a specific contagion whose properties would account for the observed phenomena. These, of course, involved much more than merely the clinical symptoms noted at the bedside. They included related aspects such as immunology and epidemiology, and in the aggregate composed the "natural history of the disease." There is, I believe, a definite analogy between the eventual discovery of the typhoid bacillus and the discovery of the planet Neptune.

THE GROWTH OF NEW ATTITUDES

Nosology was an eighteenth-century phenomenon that met the intellectual needs of physicians trying to bring order out of confusion. Nosologists, in classifying diseases, provided a series of niches or pigeonholes, each identified by its definition. The great problem was finding a suitable definition that would allow effective discrimination. Most of the data were drawn from symptoms observed directly at the bedside. The definitions and the groupings of diseases, based on available data, engendered much dispute, which manifested the rationalist trends of the eighteenth century.

The whole mental set changed when physicians began to evaluate diseases in terms of total patterns rather than in terms of concise definitions. The process, of course, involves nothing less than the massive transformation of thought modes, and this is precisely what took place in the first half of the nineteenth century.

I can mention here only a few of the operative factors. There was a deliberate search for new data and new relationships, a process now called research. During the early nineteenth century, these new data came principally from morbid anatomy, which showed a clear and direct relevance to clinical findings. The sciences of chemistry and physiology also made great progress, but their relevance to clinical problems was a little more remote and took more time to become operative. They did influence medical theory but more slowly than did morbid anatomy. Advances in technology, of course, held tremendous and increasing importance throughout the century.

In the 1830s and 1840s, the essential fevers illustrate especially well this progress. The enlargement of the total data base (largely through morbid anatomy) permitted sharper discrimination of patterns among disease entities. The importance of causal agents was increasingly recognized, as physicians tried to achieve a real specificity for diseases. The path, however, was devious.

EARLY ANATOMICAL CORRELATIONS

In the early nineteenth century, when the Anglo-American views on typhus were rather confused, French physicians were providing fresh insights. In 1813 M. A. Petit (1762–1840) and E. R. A. Serres (1786–1868) published a monograph that described clinical and anatomical findings in an epidemic that attacked Paris during the preceding two years.[2] These authors observed alterations in the lower ileum, where oval areas showed changes varying from mild swelling to marked ulceration. They were attending to the lymphoid aggregates, or Peyer's patches, and the ulcerations that we now know characterize typhoid fever. They also called attention to the swollen mesenteric lymph glands.

Under the name of enteromesenteric fever, Petit and Serres lumped together all the cases that showed any changes in the lower ileum and adjacent lymph nodes. This new name certainly included cases of modern typhoid fever, and the authors deserve great credit for their descriptions. However, many of the cases they called enteromesenteric fever were probably not typhoid fever at all, for the authors lacked knowledge of the normal lymphoid aggregates and the variations that might occur therein under various conditions. Petit and Serres produced what might be called a first approximation of the anatomical changes in typhoid fever.

The authors claimed that enteromesenteric fever had its initial site in the abdomen. Admitting difficulty in explaining how the fever arose, they suggested two possible mechanisms. One involved the nervous system, stimulated by the irritation present in the abdomen. The alternative was a "material agent [*principe matériel*] that penetrates the mass of solids and fluids" and produced the symptoms. Then the question arose, What was this *principe*? Where did it come from and how did it multiply? The authors suggested that the material came from the intestine. It was a deleterious substance, of unknown nature, absorbed by the lymphatics, carried into the mass of humors, and then infecting the entire economy. The propagation occurred from the intestine into the nodes of the mesentery (ibid., pp. 160–62).

The authors considered the intestinal alteration to be the cause. The fever was not simply of nervous origin but was supported (*entretenue*) by a deleterious substance introduced into the economy. This agent (*principe*) spread first to the mesenteric glands and then infected the solids and fluids (pp. 164–65). Such concepts offered a marked contrast to the theories that Cullen had propounded.

The work of Petit and Serres was part of the French movement of clinicopathological correlations that had yielded such brilliant results with tuberculosis and other pulmonary diseases.[3] The studies on enteromesenteric fever, published at the height of the Napoleonic wars, probably had little direct influence in Great Britain and none at all in the United States. The indirect influence, however, was great.

Physicians, depending entirely on clinical symptoms, described many different "diseases" with many different names, such as putrid fever, adynamic fever, slow fever, and the like. Cullen, we have seen, considered them all synonyms of typhus, but this did not settle the question of whether the conditions were really identical. On purely clinical grounds, there was no way to tell. When, however, clinical findings could be correlated with a pattern of morbid anatomical changes, new possibilities for analysis appeared.

COMPREHENSIVE ANALYSIS: PIERRE BRETONNEAU

Pierre Bretonneau (1771–1852), a French provincial physician, greatly advanced the knowledge of typhus. He is best known, perhaps, for his identification of diphtheria in 1826. His important work on (bacterial) typhus grew out of the epidemics at Tours that began about 1816. With a precision much greater than that of Petit and Serres, he described the clinical pattern as well as the changes in the ileum and the mesenteric lymph nodes. To the disease he gave the name *dothinetérie,* transliterated into English as dothinenteritis. This neologism, coming from two Greek words meaning abscess (or pustule) and intestine, expresses reasonably well the essential morbid anatomy.

Manuscripts describing Bretonneau's findings were completed in 1822, with subsequent revisions by 1827, but were never published. His ideas, however, were widely disseminated in Paris by his pupils, especially Armand Trousseau and A. A. L. M. Velpeau. In 1922 the unpublished manuscripts were printed and made directly available for the first time.[4] His concepts had no immediate influence on American medicine, but by the 1830s were already familiar to progressive American physicians.

Nathan Smith had considered typhus a specific entity, sui generis and contagious, with immunity conferred by a single attack. Smith had no knowledge of anatomical changes but relied entirely on clinical and epidemiological evidence. Bretonneau, with much more clinical material and aided by extensive anatomical studies, reached his conclusion independently, but from his evidence he drew much more sophisticated conclusions.

In his search for specificity, Bretonneau dispensed with the term *typhus,* which Armstrong had reduced to a mere catchall, with no differential value. When Bretonneau identified a characteristic pattern within a large group of febrile diseases, a new name emphasized its uniqueness.

In claiming that the disease was contagious, Bretonneau relied not only on analogy but also on the study of epidemics. Contagion was hard to prove on purely clinical grounds, yet when dothinenteritis appeared suddenly at a single locality, and then spread gradually from house to house, from village to village, the inference of contagion seemed inescapable. He developed the parallel to exanthemata at great length.[5]

To study the broader problem of specificity, Bretonneau analyzed inflammation, together with comparable reactions in animals and plants. The essential nature of inflammation remained unknown, but he described various characteristic patterns, which differed in appearance and development according to the stimulus. He offered many examples to correlate particular agents and particular reactions. He pointed to the distinct lesions of scabies, ringworm, and yaws in humans, and to the various excrescences produced by particular insects acting on plants. Different agents could modify the vital properties in special and characteristic fashion (ibid., pp. 336–38).

In all this he was calling attention to patterns of reaction, each distinguishable from the others if observed with sufficient care. Specificity seemed to mean a stability of pattern that, despite variations in time and place, remained both constant and identifiable.

Then he went on to discuss specificity of cause. Many disorders, especially inflammations, "are determined by material extrinsic causes, by real entities [*veritables êtres*] coming from without, or at least, foreign to the normal state of organic structure" (p. 342). That these agents were alive he emphasized by using the term *entozoa*—living entities (*êtres vivants*). They could reproduce.

Variola, for example, had for its source (*principe*) an entity capable of reproduction that united itself to the pustular matter. Variola as a disease could not be regarded merely as an inflammation, the simple result of an active agent. Instead, the disease resulted from the presence of the agent throughout the entire bodily economy. The pustular eruption was only one manifestation. Even though the local symptoms could be allayed, the patient might die from hidden effects of the variolous essence (*être varioloque*) (pp. 342–43).

In scarlatina, considered to be another exanthem, the patient might die without any observable visceral lesions. In such a case, the patient succumbed "to the effects of a poison introduced into the economy, with the remarkable property of multiplying there, to become a new focus of infection, and to cause death without leaving any other trace of its activity than a superficial inflammation of the pharynx and skin" (p. 343). Clearly, Bretonneau had firmly grasped the concept of infectious agents, invisible but self-reproducing, each producing its own distinctive pattern and therefore specific.

Furthermore, this concept of specificity he applied to any inflammatory process that showed a definite and characteristic course and also could be transmitted from one individual to another. The disease dothinenteritis manifested in the highest degree the characters of a specific inflammation. It showed an exanthematous type of inflammation, a regular progression in development, and a transmissibility, or at least a tendency to epidemic propagation. Furthermore, this disease differed strikingly from other inflammatory conditions affecting the intestine, such as dysentery or tuberculosis. And finally, those who had the disease were extremely unlikely to contract it a second time (pp. 348–57).

While emphasizing the specificity of dothinenteritis, Bretonneau admitted that he could not explain how the pustular eruption in the intestine could be fatal. However, he could point to many other diseases, including rabies, tetanus, or strychnine poisoning, where, after death, no appreciable lesion could be found. Inability to provide an explanation meant that "the special and essential quality of the inflammation has a quite different significance than the intensity." Furthermore, "the specificity of many morbid affections is their most important characteristic" (p. 330).

Bretonneau, by insisting on specificity, stressed the qualitative aspects of pathology. He vigorously rejected reductionism, whereby differences in kind would be attributed to varying degrees of a single pathological activity—the doctrine that Southwood Smith was then advocating. A qualitative approach emphasized distinct patterns, each of which included the clinical course, anatomical findings, epidemiologic data, and whatever was known about immunology.

The patterns showed stability under various circumstances and did not get confused one with another. Particular agents could not ordinarily be demonstrated, but they were postulated to account for the observed effects. The isolation of responsible living agents would be the work of the future.

Nathan Smith and Pierre Bretonneau, thousands of miles apart and practicing under markedly different conditions, came to surprisingly similar conclusions. Bretonneau enjoyed much deeper knowledge and greater professional advantages, and he carried his work much further forward than did the American, but the insistence on patterns and specificity reveal similar insights, achieved independently.

PIERRE LOUIS AND THE NUMERICAL METHOD

The third major contribution from France came from Pierre Louis (1787–1872), whose methodology helped to transform the methods of medical science. In 1829 Louis published his important study of typhoid fever. His book, compiling masses of unassailable data, bore the informative title, *Recherches anatomiques, pathologiques et thérapeutiques sur la maladie connue sous les noms de gastro-entérite, fièvre putride, adynamique, ataxique, typhoide, etc. etc. Comparée avec les maladies aigues les plus ordinaires.*[6]

Shortly after publication in France the book received in the United States a long and highly laudatory essay review, which summarized the contents in detail.[7] Louis's book was in four parts. The first described minutely the histories of eighteen fatal cases in which both symptoms and anatomical lesions were well developed. The second studied anatomical changes in fatal cases and also in controls dying of other acute diseases. The analysis firmly established the "anatomical characteristic" of the disease. Then Louis compared the symptoms of those who had died of "typhus" and those who had recovered. The controls and the analysis enabled him to distinguish conclusively between the essential and the accidental features in the disease. And finally he examined the data relative to therapy.

The total amount of detail is staggering. The reviewer commented on "an indefatigability of investigation, a niceness of discrimination, a faithfulness of delineation, and an exactness of deduction which cannot be too much admired nor too closely imitated." He praised the work highly, declaring it a "model of medical research, worthy of imitation." From the work, "a flood of light would beam upon medical science" and would "enlighten many parts of it, now apparently enveloped in almost impenetrable darkness. The present era," said the reviewer, could now "place medical science upon the firm bases of correct observation, critical research, and strict philosophical deduction . . . [and] discard all speculation and vain hypotheses."

Quite significantly, however, the reviewer constantly referred to the disease as "typhus," regardless of Louis's nomenclature. Furthermore, the reviewer said nothing of the specificity of disease nor the effect the book might have on the classification of fevers. These problems had not made much impression on most American physicians of the period.

If we compare this work of Louis with that of Petit and Serres published only half a generation earlier, we note a striking difference in method. Petit and Serres had tried to differentiate their enteromesenteric fever from conditions previously described under such names as adynamic fever, ataxic fever, and mucous fever.[8] Differences certainly existed, but how constantly? Were they essential or merely accidental? How much overlap between the different conditions? On these questions Petit and Serres could not provide rigorous evidence. Louis's methods, however, enabled him to give convincing answers and to show that the different names were really the same disease entity. Petit and Serres had regarded enteromesenteric fever "as a link that unites these three species of fever" (p. 170). Louis, however, showed their identity.

Yet Louis's book on typhoid fever had certain defects that have generally been passed over. Debreuil-Chambardel criticized him for ignoring Bretonneau. To be sure, the latter had not himself published anything on the subject. But his students had, and his doctrines had been vigorously discussed in Paris. Furthermore, Louis did not recognize the contagious nature of the disease nor perceive that a living being, comparable to the entozoa, was the causal agent. Bretonneau had much more mental acuity and insight than Louis and perceived a more comprehensive pattern. He was by far the greater investigator.

Louis's book had little direct effect on American medicine. A translation was not published in the United States until 1836, and reviews did little to spread new ideas.[9] Louis' influence was exerted in this country less by the written word than by the physicians who went to France, trained there, and then returned to this country to practice.

WILLIAM GERHARD AND SHARP DISCRIMINATION

The first three decades of the nineteenth century threw much light on the so-called essential fevers, but many obscurities remained. The British and the French used the same word, *typhus,* but they did not necessarily refer to the same entity. In Great Britain, only some of the cases called typhus showed at autopsy the ulcerations that the French pathologists found. Were British typhus and French typhus separate diseases or simply varieties of the same disease? Were there transitions between the two? At what point could we distinguish a basic difference in kind from a mere difference in degree? Could ulceration of the ileum serve as a strict criterion for diagnosis? In solving these problems of specificity, American physicians played a major part, and of them William Gerhard (1809–72) deserves special credit.[10]

Gerhard had an excellent educational background. A graduate of Dickinson College in 1826, he served an apprenticeship and received his M.D. degree from the University of Pennsylvania in 1830. The years 1831–33 he spent abroad, mostly in Paris working under Louis.

In the United States at that time there were relatively few hospitals, and these were small compared with the huge French institutions. Most of Gerhard's research was done at the Pennsylvania Hospital, which had about fifty beds exclusively for medical patients. The number of medical cases varied between 300 and 400 a year. Medical patients included many sailors from merchant vessels that stopped in the port of Philadelphia as well as "mechanics and laborers" from the city and its environs. Because of the large number of sailors admitted, the physicians saw many diseases not ordinarily observed in charity hospitals drawing only on the local population.

Most of the care was given by two resident physicians, who alternated between the medical and the surgical wards. For the most part, these residents were "very young men who have but just entered upon the duties of the physician, or have not yet completed their preliminary duties." Gerhard, however, after his long training with Louis, knew that "the art of observation requires a long apprenticeship; he who has not passed through the period of preparation is not capable of observing facts, still less of making any useful deductions from them."[11]

In 1835, as resident physician, he wrote his first paper on typhus. Was the disease called typhus in Philadelphia the same as that which he had studied in Paris as typhoid fever? In his paper Gerhard used the terms *typhus fever* (the typhus of other authors) and *typhoid fever* quite interchangeably.

In an eight-month period in 1834, sixty-two patients entered the hospital with a diagnosis of fever, of whom fourteen were considered to have typhus or typhoid fever. Of these fourteen patients, five died; autopsies were performed on two of the five. The postmortem findings revealed the typical lesions of the ileum, abdominal lymph nodes, and spleen that characterized the typhoid fever of Louis. In contrast, two autopsied cases of remittent fever showed markedly different anatomical findings. Gerhard concluded that typhus in Philadelphia was identical with the typhoid fever that Louis had described in Paris.

Gerhard had not as yet come to grips with the problem of whether the typhoid fever of Louis (occurring also in Philadelphia) was the same as what the British called typhus. Opportunity for such a comparison occurred in 1836, when a severe epidemic became manifest in Philadelphia. The disease differed from the bilious fever, yellow fever, and other "malignant intermittents," but resembled the typhus of Great Britain and Ireland that had been much described (and which we now know is due to a rickettsia). It also resembled the 1813 epidemics in France and Philadelphia (the latter causing the death of Benjamin Rush). A Philadelphia physician who had lived through that epidemic, and who also saw the cases occurring in 1836, immediately recognized the similarity.[12]

For the current epidemic, Gerhard wanted "to ascertain if there was a real fundamental difference between the form of disease which prevailed . . . and the dothinenteritis [Gerhard was obviously familiar with Bretonneau's work], which is always to be met with in America as a sporadic affection." The crucial term here is *fundamental,* whose meaning will fluctuate with the bias of the observer. What one person considers fundamental, another might regard as incidental.

Gerhard's approach to the problem reflected the training he had received from Louis. He studied autopsy findings, symptoms, mode of communication, and treatment. And at each step he made comparisons with dothinenteritis. Moreover, he clarified the nomenclature. The British typhus seemed to be the same disease that earlier physicians had called typhus gravior, ship fever, jail fever, camp fever, and petechial or spotted fever. The dothinenteritis or typhoid fever of the French was the same as typhus mitior. And, he might have added, as the typhous fever of Nathan Smith.

Gerhard's papers dealt in part with anatomical findings and

overall pattern, in part with clinical symptoms The (rickettsial) typhus showed no constant morbid changes of the internal organs, and he emphasized the differences from typhoid fever, which regularly involved the ileum, spleen, and lymph nodes. In (rickettsial) typhus the most constant anatomical change was the cutaneous eruption, found in thirty-two of thirty-six white patients, and clearly different from the skin eruption of typhoid fever. He classed typhus with the exanthemata, which also showed no constant morbid change apart from the cutaneous eruptions.

The skin lesions of typhoid fever and of typhus were as readily distinguishable, he said, as those of measles and smallpox. There was strong evidence that typhus was transmitted by direct contagion. Gerhard gave many examples of spread from one patient to another and from patients to attending nurses and physicians. However, since the disease had appeared in widely scattered parts of Philadelphia, it was not possible to trace direct connections between the different foci. He could not point to any single discrete etiologic agent but thought that some "general cause" was also acting. Among the factors that helped to spread the disease, he mentioned poverty, overcrowding, race, age, occupation, and the season of the year.

To distinguish (British or rickettsial) typhus from typhoid fever, Gerhard provided detailed clinical histories, together with autopsy protocols that we must still regard as excellent. He also analyzed the symptoms and the differential features. The proper diagnosis required "a careful examination of the symptoms presented during life, and of the phenomena observed after death." If the symptoms and the lesions occurred together with sufficient frequency, they would then permit a "generalization."[13]

Phenomena came not singly but in groups and clusters or, in Gerhard's word, in "series." Physicians needed to observe the character and intensity of symptoms at different periods and note whether a series, or succession of phenomena, was "nearly, if not quite, constant. If this series does occur in the large majority of cases," then the symptoms showed a relation "sufficiently constant for us to admit them as constituting a distinct disease." If not all but only the most important symptoms were present, then the absence of the others "does not materially impair the diagnosis" (ibid.).

These statements embody important concepts. Gerhard's concern with series and relationship reveals his keen appreciation of pattern in the understanding of disease. The disease was not a loose aggregate of separate symptoms, but the symptoms, through some inner connection, hung together in a constant pattern. Different aspects, which included the temporal course, cohered. His critics did not grasp this sense of an inner connection but regarded the individual features as if they were in isolation.

In the early stages, Gerhard pointed out, typhoid and typhus fevers did resemble each other, but no more than did the early stages of typhoid fever and smallpox. Typhoid fever (for which he often used as synonym Bretonneau's term *dothinenteritis*) was a sporadic disease, although it occasionally appeared in epidemics; typhus was primarily an epidemic disease, rarely sporadic. Typhus was very contagious; typhoid fever was not, under ordinary circumstances. Gerhard offered many other clinical contrasts, not necessary to recount here. Although some cases would remain doubtful, he was defining patterns that could separate most cases of continued fever into distinct entities.

Today we fully appreciate Gerhard's work in establishing typhoid fever and typhus as two distinct and specific diseases, but his papers exerted little immediate influence. While he found a few strong supporters for the specificity of each disease, many writers were not convinced.

The earliest major support I could find occurred in the American edition of a British textbook by Marshall Hall.[14] The "First American Edition, revised and much enlarged by Jacob Bigelow and Oliver Wendell Holmes" was published in Boston in 1839. The portions rewritten by the American authors (always clearly indicated) included an excellent discussion of typhoid and typhus fevers. There is a fine account of recent scientific contributions. Bigelow and Holmes favorably analyzed Gerhard's work and fully accepted it.

A VIGOROUS SUPPORTER OF GERHARD: ELISHA BARTLETT

Even more influential was Elisha Bartlett's text on fevers, *The History, Diagnosis, and Treatment of Fevers in the United States*, originally published in 1843, with an expanded second edition in

1847.[15] Bartlett (1804–55) fully supported Gerhard, and discussed many of the significant problems. For example, he did not believe that the lesions in the ileum "were the local cause of all the other appreciable phenomena of typhoid fever" but were "themselves the result of some morbific agent, or influence, or process" (ibid. p. 832). Typhoid fever was a specific infection, differing from a "common" infection such as bronchitis. The latter disease was highly variable in character, the former was not. He, too, held that the lesions in the ileum had the same relation to typhoid fever that in smallpox the skin pustules had to its disease. The ileal lesions were specific and could not be induced "at will by any of the ordinary excitants of common inflammation" (p. 139).

Bartlett distinguished between the individual symptoms, or the typhoid state, and the disease of typhoid fever. As a modern paraphrase, a pattern as a whole must be distinguished from its components. Only the whole pattern was specific, the individual elements were not. Some *typhoid phenomena . . . are often present in many diseases* such as peritonitis, pneumonia, erysipelas, and dysentery. Such phenomena were not to be "confounded with typhoid fever, the specific disease" (p. 132).

After discussing typhoid fever, Bartlett made a comparable analysis for typhus. Here, however, his personal experience was limited and he had to rely largely on the literature. He considered typhus a contagious disease, appearing in epidemics, especially under conditions of poverty, filth, and overcrowding. "The poison of typhus fever is generated in a stagnant and depraved atmosphere, rank with the thick corruptions of concentrated emanations from the living human body." Typhoid fever "is generated as readily amidst cleanliness and purity as amidst filth" (p. 243).

If the diseases were distinct, they must be distinguishable on clinical grounds. Bartlett listed twelve clinical features (apart from the anatomical lesions) that might serve as differential points. He laid particular stress on the differences between the rose spots of typhoid fever and the petechial eruption found in typhus (pp. 274–75).

In 1848 Bartlett's book received a long and detailed review.[16] The reviewer declared that on clinical grounds the two diseases were often indistinguishable, and concluded "that the typhoid is a mere form or variety of the typhus fever." If the anatomical changes were an essential distinction, the relation of lesions and symptoms must, he said, be invariable. But some cases, with all the clinical features of typhoid fever, did not show lesions. These, however, might occur in other cases lacking the characteristic clinical findings. The reviewer believed it was "much safer to consider the typhoid as one of the forms of typhus fever." The evidence that Gerhard, Bartlett, and others had provided made little impression on the reviewer.

VIGOROUS OPPONENTS OF GERHARD

Another disagreement with Gerhard's concepts came from the American Medical Association. Its precursor, the National Medical Association, meeting in 1847, had appointed a committee to report on the latest developments in "practical medicine." A year later, at the first meeting of the new American Medical Association, the report was tendered by Joseph M. Smith (1789–1866).[17] Smith had served as surgeon's mate in the War of 1812 and then received his M.D. degree in 1815 from the New York College of Physicians and Surgeons. In his long career he had gained considerable experience with epidemics, a field in which he was widely accepted as an authority.

Smith's report provided interesting details of the typhus epidemics that accompanied the great immigrations, especially from famine-stricken Ireland. For Smith, the disease did not arise from "a specific contagious principle" comparable to that of smallpox. Rather, the poison came from chemical changes "in the excretions or *debris* of the body . . . accumulated in close apartments." It was "generated by the exhalations and other excretive matters of typhus patients" more readily than by patients suffering from other diseases.[18] The human body, he thought, could give rise to the infectious principle of typhus, de novo, in any filthy environment.

Smith disagreed with the "renowned pathologists" who held that typhoid fever and typhus were essentially different. In maintaining the opposite, he asked two cogent questions. Were the symptoms such that physicians could characterize them as "distinct distempers"? Did the evidence from morbid anatomy indicate that the diseases were "specifically different"?

Clinical features that Smith claimed occurred in both typhus and typhoid fever included some that Bartlett said occurred chiefly in only one. Smith rejected any data opposed to his own claims. If, he said, the two diseases were "specifically different," they should "present certain pathognomonic or characteristic symptoms" (ibid., p. 118). He refused to accept the skin eruption as a differential point. "To elevate the shades of colour, and the varieties of the form of the eruption to the rank of diagnostic phenomena, indicative of distinct diseases, when the more striking and important phenomena are unequivocally expressive of an identity . . . is a refinement . . . no clinical observer can regard with favour" (p. 120).

After declaring that individual symptoms would not suffice to separate typhoid fever from typhus, Smith turned to "general symptomatology." The various idiopathic fevers he distinguished "by the kind and character of their general symptoms" and by the ways these developed. The diagnosis would rest "on the type, and the general course and peculiarity of the phenomena manifested in the nervous, vascular, and secretory functions" (pp. 121–22). He depended not on carefully studied patterns, such as Nathan Smith and Gerhard had offered, but on vague impressions that he could not support with precise evidence.

When comparing the two diseases, he declared in turgid prose, "the morbid phenomena are so correspondent in the sensorial, vascular and other functions, and are so similarly catenated" that attempts to make then into "two different diseases . . . must fail to show any distinction which is found in nature and recognizable by practical minds" (p. 122). Clearly, practical minds differed from scientific minds.

The work of Gerhard could not be ignored but could be explained away. Smith thought that "the differences in morbid anatomy of the two epidemics . . . were due to incidental causes; and that the two epidemics were the same disease modified in different seasons" (p. 130). What Gerhard considered essential, Smith dismissed as mere incidental variation. He did not see the significance of clinicopathological correlation. He wanted to isolate clinical symptoms from anatomical changes. For Gerhard, Bartlett, and other younger men, clinical and anatomical changes formed part of a total natural history, a total gestalt or pattern, distinct for each disease. Smith could not grasp this concept. Even in 1850, he was bogged down in eighteenth-century thinking, seeking individual clinical symptoms that would be pathognomonic for a disease.

Henry F. Campbell (1824–91) came to Joseph Smith's conclusion by a different route.[19] Campbell headed a three-man committee appointed to study the "typhoidal diseases." Campbell, thirty-five years younger than Smith, attended the Medical College of Georgia, graduating in 1842 when he was only eighteen years of age. He practiced in Georgia for most of his life. In his special fields, surgery and gynecology, he achieved considerable prominence. In 1884 he was president of the AMA.

When in 1853 he wrote on typhoidal fevers, he could not have had much personal clinical experience. He based his analysis on the data of others and provided an explanation through "rational induction." He wanted merely to "interpret" the "facts" already recorded. Relying on the data of others would "be less liable to fallacy" than if he merely interpreted his own cases, "always liable to preconceived opinions and forgone conclusions" (ibid., 421–22). This reference to "preconceived opinions" is worth keeping in mind.

Campbell did not minimize the differences between typhoid fever and typhus, nor did he search for diagnostic criteria. Both diseases belonged to the inclusive category, typhoidal fevers, for which he wanted to find a single cause. He also tried to identify factors that would explain the observed differences between the two conditions. The pronounced changes in the intestine he regarded as secondary to something still more primary, from which both the lesions and the symptoms derived. He was seeking an overall explanation, which he called the "ultimate pathology" (p. 448).

Typhus and typhoid fever, he said, were "at least *similar* and even by many considered *identical*." The symptoms centered around the nervous system, the circulation, and the digestive system. The same systems were involved in both typhoid fever and typhus, but not with the same intensity. Yet the one disease exhibited marked intestinal lesions, the other did not. "Now it would be very surprising if two sets of symptoms [i.e., the two diseases], so exactly simulating each other, that the most skillful and experienced have denied the least difference between them, should arise from entirely different causes. . . . Certainly such a conclusion would not be very philosophical" (p. 453).

The words, "exactly simulating" of course, completely beg the question, intruding his preexisting conclusions into his data, and blandly assuming what demanded rigorous proof. The two diseases had features in common but also differences. Admitting this, Campbell regarded the similarities as important and the differences as insignificant.

He continued with his *petitio principi*. Typhoid fever, he said, had "its unmistakable counterpart . . . typhus fever." These two diseases are "inseparably bound together in ties of the strongest and most indissoluble affinity." If a theory entails the necessity of separating the two diseases, this "is enough, of itself, to declare its absurdity" (p. 454). Any disagreement with the author thus was, a priori, absurd.

In spite of his arrogant dogmatism, Campbell's reasoning is worth examining. For Campbell, basic pathology lay in the sympathetic nervous system, with its prevertebral chain and the visceral ganglia. The ganglionic system "controls the important acts of circulation, secretion, and nutrition; or at least, forms a necessary element in these functions." And the symptoms of typhoid fever were located in the organs innervated by the ganglionic system (p. 461).

Surgical experiments that interfered with the sympathetic system produced numerous physiological disturbances. With these results, some of the phenomena in typhoid fever showed "a close analogy, if not identity." He concluded that the typhoid phenomena "are but the result of aberration in the normal action" of the sympathetic nervous system (pp. 461–68). The word *but* reveals the extreme reductionism that I call the "nothing-but" fallacy.

Typhoid fever and typhus "have all their general symptoms so exactly similar that we are forced to acknowledge their identity, and see in them what is essentially one disease." Typhoid fever involved principally the abdominal viscera. Typhus "manifests itself in aberrations of the circulation, very analogous to those of typhoid, but occurring in the capillaries of the *cutaneous* surface." In typhoid fever and typhus, then, "*the disease is one and the same*, but seated in different portions of the organism." The "morbific agent" affected different nerve centers in the two conditions, in typhus the sympathetic (prevertebral) chain, in typhoid fever the visceral ganglia (pp. 470–71). The minutiae of the explanation need not concern us.

Campbell admitted it would be better if he could show some actual lesions in the ganglia, but the absence of anatomic changes was easily explained. Alterations were probably "molecular and inappreciable with our present means of investigation." Time and "more perfect appliances" (i.e., better technology) would be needed (p. 472). Lack of evidence did not concern him. Presumably there, it simply was not yet observable.

All this is a truly virtuoso performance in the worst of eighteenth-century thinking. Campbell started with "the vast number of reliable and significant facts," which all showed the identity of typhus (now sometimes called typhus fever or genuine typhus) and typhoid fever. When these "well-ascertained facts" were "rationally and correctly *interpreted*" (p. 474), they proved (to Campbell) that both diseases resulted from disturbed action of the sympathetic nervous system. Discordant evidence had been rejected in advance.

THE MODERN CRITICAL ATTITUDE: AUSTIN FLINT

In marked contrast to Campbell was Austin Flint. He received his M.D. degree from Harvard in 1832. Although he never studied in France, some of his medical school teachers had come under the French influence and helped to form his thinking in the newer mode. In 1836 he went to Buffalo, New York, where he achieved an excellent reputation. Eventually he went to New York City, where he soon became an outstanding clinician and educator. Among his many honors was the presidency of the AMA in 1883. His textbook on the principles and practice of medicine went through six editions during his lifetime and one posthumously.[20] His name survives in the Austin Flint murmur of the heart.

In 1843, in a small New York community eighteen miles from Buffalo, a baffling epidemic induced local physicians to call on Flint for help. His report was a truly masterful study.[21] The epidemic started when a young man, traveling westward and finding himself ill, stopped at the local tavern. There he died, some four weeks later. Members of the tavern-keeper's family soon became ill, and the disease spread to nearby households, with several deaths.

The febrile symptoms differed from those of the prevalent "mild remittent or bilious fever" familiar to local physicians. One physician thought the disease was a remittent fever that showed irregular remissions and "putrid or typhoid symptoms." For Flint, however, the clinical findings, supported by autopsy, showed "clearly" that the disease was the same as that prevailing in New England. This, in turn, was the same as Louis had described in France as typhoid fever. Flint traced the origin of the present epidemic to the stranger who had come from New England (where the disease was common) and who died twenty-three days before the next case appeared. The spread then became more rapid. For Flint, the epidemic proved the contagiousness of typhoid fever. The stranger had presumably left New England "with the germinal principle of typhoid fever in his system."

Flint noted the distinction between the typhoid state or "typhoid symptoms," which local physicians had observed, and typhoid fever, which Flint regarded as a distinct disease. He raised the further question, whether typhoid fever and typhus were two distinct forms of fever or "only modifications of the same form." In his account of the event, he declined to take up the question, but he did return to it several years later.

For many years, he amassed data on typhoid fever and published much of it in journals. His important text on continued fever, published in 1852, reprinted these journal articles, while new material explained his methodology and the way in which he critically evaluated evidence.[22] It was an excellent contribution to the logic of medicine and scientific method.

In the class of continued fever, Flint recognized two separable forms, typhus and typhoid fever. To distinguish them, physicians would need to compare respective symptoms and pathological findings. Yet even before they could make such a comparison and identify similar or dissimilar features, they first would have to make an initial discrimination according to some criteria. Hence, data collected according to these criteria would, in a sense, be preselected.

Typhoid fever and typhus showed many features in common but also many differences. Some differences were only a matter of degree, but there were also important qualitative differences. Of these Flint noted especially the skin eruptions observed during life and the anatomical changes in the ileum found at autopsy. Louis had asserted that anatomical lesions in the ileum, spleen, and lymph nodes were criteria for distinguishing typhoid fever from typhus, yet other physicians had claimed that these anatomical lesions were also found in typhus. This latter allegation was used to support the identity of the two diseases. Obviously, the same lesion occurring in both diseases could not serve to differentiate between them.

Flint referred to his own extensive experience. He had noted intestinal lesions in twelve autopsied cases. Of these, nine had been diagnosed during life as typhoid fever, and three as typhus. In the latter cases, however, the changes in the Peyer's patches were very slight, and quite insignificant when compared with those in typhoid fever. Flint concluded that in cases clinically diagnosed as typhus, the follicles (the Peyer's patches) "do not always continue wholly unaffected." Yet the character of the changes in the typhus cases differed markedly from what was observed in cases diagnosed as typhoid fever during life (ibid., pp. 240–41).

Any claim that lesions in the ileum occurred in typhus, and therefore were not specific for typhoid fever, had to face two questions: How accurate were the observations? and How reliable was the observer? Especially important here was the allegation of a French clinician (identified only by his last name, Landouzy), who described lesions in the ileum of cases of clinical typhus. His alleged observations, repeatedly mentioned, carried great weight with physicians who regarded the two diseases as essentially the same. However, there was evidence that showed how casual and haphazard was his examination and how lacking in precision.

Flint, too, questioned the accuracy of Landouzy's statements and declared "that every provision for accuracy should be required before accepting as valid, observations which conflict materially with other well-authenticated facts."[23] All observers were not equal. Flint emphasized the need for critical evaluation of proferred evidence.

He raised a further point in methodology. Anatomical changes, which could vary in degree and character, could not by themselves provide the criterion for diagnosing typhoid fever. Instead, he said, "it is by the ensemble of symptoms during life that the determination of the type of fever is to be made." At any rate, "the basis of the division into the two types is the *ante-mortem* history."[24] Anatomical lesions would need to be correlated with clinical findings to help confirm or correct the diagnosis. In this way the natural history of the two diseases could be established.

Flint continued, "Do the two types possess sufficiently distinctive traits to be nosologically separated? If so, the distinction is undoubtedly . . . strengthened by the fact that certain special lesions are peculiar to one of the types." The question whether these lesions "are invariably present, is to be settled by repeated examinations after death," when the "distinctive traits" of the diseases had already been noted during life, that is, where clinical study had already indicated the type of disease (ibid., pp. 245–46). In this way, the identity or nonidentity of typhus and typhoid fever would be "fairly and fully" determined by observation.

Flint used the word *ensemble*. Present-day terminology would say that identification rested on patterns and not on pathognomonic symptoms. Patterns would be noted initially at the bedside and then expand as new data accumulated, all contributing to the "natural history" of the disease.

Unlike many of his contemporaries, Flint believed in patience before coming to a final decision. He would not commit himself on the ultimate relations of typhoid fever and typhus, and he protested strongly against the loose usage of terms. Cases with typhuslike symptoms were often called typhus or typhoid fever "without inquiring whether other essential diagnostic criteria were present or not. A *Typhoid condition* is one thing and *Typhoid fever* another" (p. 254; see also pp. 246–47). The diagnosis of typhoid fever cannot rest on the mere presence of typhoidlike symptoms. Flint thus emphasized the difference between symptoms and disease. Typhoid symptoms, such as a clouded mentation, could be the elements of a pattern, but we are not justified in asserting a whole pattern merely from observing a few of its elements.

We must admire Flint for his critical attitude, which exhibits the very best aspects of modern scientific medicine. We can sense the marked differences in modes of thinking if we compare Flint with Caldwell or Campbell. The comparison will help to characterize the distinctions between eighteenth-century thinking and that of the nineteenth century. With Austin Flint, American medicine was fully participating in the best of nineteenth-century medicine.

6

Congestive Fever and the Clinical Entity

WILLIAM CULLEN DIVIDED THE PRIMARY OR ESSEN-tial fevers into the continued and intermittent, depending on their temporal character. Unlike continued fevers, intermittents showed a periodicity, wherein febrile attacks alternated regularly with complete remission of symptoms. Physicians could make subdivisions according to the period of recurrence, as shown by the names tertian, quartan, or quotidian.

This simple division did not work very well, for many patients would not fit neatly into either schema. The periodicity might be incomplete, the febrile course would wax and wane, and while the chills might recur more or less regularly, the remissions would not be complete. Febrile symptoms would persist in the intervals between the chills, and there might be no period in which the patient was free of symptom.

REMITTENT FEVER AND ITS PLACE IN EIGHTEENTH-CENTURY NOSOLOGY

Most nosologists placed these cases in a new major group, called remittent fever, so that the essential fevers were then categorized as intermittent, remittent, or continued. In the class of remittents the patients would show exacerbations and remissions, but the remissions were not "complete." The category of remittent fever was especially important in the United States, where the malarial diseases were vastly more prevalent than in Great Britain.

By the first quarter of the nineteenth century, formal nosology, with its rigid subdivisions, was receiving less attention in medical theory. Nevertheless, some new formulations appeared in nosology, in which remittent fever received much attention. The concepts of this disease gradually developed and in so doing illustrate the transformation taking place in medical thinking in the early nineteenth century.

Formal nosology was really an eighteenth-century institution, representing, in its way, the passion for order and system, with everything in its place and a place for everything. This comprehensive view had been achieved at the expense of precision. Vague definitions had been considered satisfactory, but satisfaction lessened when physicians became more discriminating, and vagueness was seen as a defect. This change took place as newer thought modes began to make themselves felt.

Two new nosologies of the early nineteenth century deserve mention, one written by a British physician, John Mason Good (1764–1827), the other by an American, David Hosack (1769–1835). Hosack published a nosology in 1818, with a second edition in 1821.[1] Born in New York, he had received his medical training as an apprentice, but in 1791 went abroad for two years to study in Edinburgh and London. On his return to New York he soon established himself as a leading physician and surgeon, an expert in botany and mineralogy, and a prolific author. His attitudes and methods reflected those of the eighteenth century, rather than the new spirit of the nineteenth.

For the essential fevers, he adopted the groupings of intermittent, remittent, and continued. Among the intermittents he noted variation of symptoms in different cases. Some showed stupor or drowsiness, spasms or convulsions, as well as association with other diseases, such as dysentery.

The remittents Hosack defined as fevers "without perfect intermission, attended with sensible and regular exacerbations and abatements" (ibid., p. 186). Within this group he distinguished two subgroups, the bilious and the infantile. In the United States, bilious fever was a popular diagnosis. Characteristically, there were a disorder of the digestive organs and "an inordinate secretion of bile," so that the skin and eyes turned yellow. He distinguished a mild form, in which the intellectual functions were not impaired, and a malignant form, with great prostration and other ominous features ordinarily associated with typhus, including severe disturbance of the sensorium and intellectual functions.

The second subdivision of remittent fever, the infantile form, occurred in children under twelve years of age. Here the clinical features included derangement of the digestive organs, increased heat, and tendency to delirium and coma. Worm infestation was suggested as the cause. This disease conformed to the definition of remittent fever, for the symptoms showed some remission, but otherwise had little in common with the other subdivisions.

John Mason Good's writings had considerable influence in this country. In 1817 he published a nosology that provided the framework for his popular text, *The Study of Medicine*. This first appeared in 1822, with at least four British editions. By 1835 six American editions had been published, indicating the remarkable popularity of this work in the United States.[2]

Good's terminology was pedantic and idiosyncratic. He defined remittent fevers as "strikingly exacerbating and remitting, but without intermission," and divided them into three species—mild remittent, malignant remittent, and hectic fevers (ibid., vol. 2, p. 146). The latter, the type that ordinarily characterized phthisis or "consumption," was included because it conformed to his definition.

In active tuberculosis, the temperature was usually higher in the afternoon than in the morning. This phenomenon did indeed constitute an exacerbation, and there certainly was no complete intermission, that is, a period of normal temperature. Using his definition as the sole criterion, Good placed tuberculosis in the same category as intermittent fever, ignoring all the points of difference. The power of definition alone, without any sense of pattern, made strange bedfellows. We will not consider further his comments on phthisis.

In the analysis of remittent fever, his discussion of the mild remittents is noncontributory here. More significant was his second subdivision, malignant remittents. These he identified as having "pulse small, hurried, irregular; debility extreme; often with signs of putrescency." This species had four "varieties," described in considerable detail. Of most importance were the common "autumnal remittent," widely prevalent in the United States, and yellow fever. The others are not relevant here (pp. 149, 150).

Good arranged diseases according to the way they conformed (or did not conform) to a definition. If a disease showed a few points of similarity to the definition, this would establish membership in a class, regardless of the points of difference. Similarities and differences were not critically evaluated, and membership in a class was lightly asserted.

JOHN EBERLE'S DIFFERENT DISCRIMINATION

When we go from Good's textbook to the 1831 text of John Eberle, we seem to pass from the eighteenth century into the nineteenth.[3] Eberle and Good exemplify quite different modes of thinking. Eberle was not hobbled by a nosological schema into which all diseases had to fit. Instead, he provided a free-flowing exposition of diseases, took account of exceptional cases, and indicated complexities and uncertainties. His discussion of periodic fevers is quite informative.

Nosologists ordinarily separated the strict intermittents according to the interval between paroxysms, such as tertian, quartan, and the like. Eberle, however, was little concerned with periodicity but attended rather to other features that had been largely neglected. He distinguished four different clinical forms of intermittents (see ibid., vol. 1, pp. 73–75). The inflammatory form occurred mostly in young and robust patients, who reacted vigorously to the disease. The rigors (i.e., the chills) were strong, the fever generally high, the pulse hard and full. Between paroxysms, headache, cough, and other symptoms might remain, so that the intermission need not be quite complete.

A second type of intermittent fever Eberle called congestive. This, although occurring but seldom, contrasted sharply with the inflammatory form. The congestive form tended "to attack persons of exhausted and debilitated habits, and . . . of an irritable and nervous temperament." The symptoms, too, were rather different. There was a long, protracted cold stage. The hot stage came on very slowly and developed "very imperfectly, so that instead of hot skin, flushed countenance, and a full and vigorous pulse, the system continued to be oppressed, the skin scarcely warm, the countenance pale and contracted, the breathing confined and anxious, and the pulse frequent, small, and tense."

A third type, the gastric intermittent, was prevalent in temperate climates. Prominent were symptoms of gastric and intestinal "irritation," often accompanied by jaundice, thirst, and "induration" of the spleen and liver. A fourth type, the malignant intermittent, was more frequent in hot (rather than merely temperate) climates and included "colliquative hemorrhages from various parts of the body, sometimes petechia [sic], and other marks of malignity." The intervals between paroxysms seemed much less important than the physiological reactions of the patients. This approach tended to break down the distinction between intermittent and remittent fevers and to direct attention to broader relationships.

For the category of remittent fever, Eberle presented first the common form, popularly called bilious fever, remarkably similar to some intermittents. "Between the simple autumnal *remittent* and *intermittent* fevers, there exists no essential or radical difference. They are produced by the same cause, and differ from each other only in the grade of violence and duration of the paroxysms" (p. 97). He emphasized that no form of fever "is subject to so great a diversity." Any description of this disease would have no more than a "very general application." Ignoring any rigid framework of genera and species, Eberle presented broad overall patterns. His presentation makes us appreciate the groping for new information, and the reevaluation of older data. He was helping to forge new attitudes as well as to find new evidence.

Remittent fever was especially dangerous in hot climates. Eberle described the intense thirst, violent headache, marked vomiting, and progressive jaundice. The severity of the symptoms would moderate during remissions but would then recur. Sometimes, he said, the urine was dark brown, sometimes entirely suppressed. The stools might be bloody. The disease, he pointed out, tended "to fall, with especial violence, on some one organ or structure, as the brain, the liver, the alimentary canal, or the blood vessels, and to assume, in consequence, a peculiar character" (p. 100). In retrospect we realize that he was probably describing infection by the virulent plasmodium falciparum, which contrasted with the more benign species of plasmodium. His descriptions suggest aspects of so-called blackwater fever.

In the hepatic form there was no bile in the vomitus, but there was a very yellow color to the skin. These features indicated a "strong manifestation of *sanguineous engorgement* and *functional inactivity of the liver*" (p. 101). In these cases, the mucosa of the stomach and bowels was "in a state of considerable irritation, and probably often of inflammation." But even more important were the inferred hepatic changes. He felt that the functional disorder of the liver "constitutes one of the most constant local affections of remitting fever" (p. 102). Yet despite his grasp of clinical manifestations and their significance, Eberle apparently did not perform any autopsies.

The epidemic form of remittent fever had as its cause the miasma rising from the soil. For this exhalation, commonly called malaria, Eberle himself preferred the term *koniomiasma*, a neologism that never caught on. This agent affected many people at one time and thus could give rise to epidemics, yet it did not spread by contact. In contrast, the effluvium (which he called *idiomiasma*), "originating from the decomposition of matter derived from the human body," was truly contagious—that is, it could transmit the disease directly from one person to another (pp. 45–50). William Cullen, we recall, had made a comparable separation of causes.

Other causes might produce symptoms of remittent fever. "Worms and other irritating substances lodged in the bowels, may give rise to a regularly remitting form of fever," often known as "infantile remittent," but in this form the biliary organs were less likely to be involved.

Whatever the cause, the principal "morbid irritation" always affected the abdominal organs, especially the liver and the mucosa of the intestinal tract. For Eberle the term *gastric fever* seemed preferable to the more usual *remittent fever,* "which has no reference to the pathological condition of the system" (p. 104). To a considerable extent, he was thinking in terms of physiology, pathology, and etiology. His analysis deserves the title physiological medicine far more than did the effusions of Broussais.

Even without anatomical studies, Eberle's emphasis on pathology represents an important insight. The usual classification, he realized, might juxtapose diseases that were quite distinct, and he gave hectic fever as an example. Good classed this disease with the remittents, for the temperature swing seemed to fit the definition of remittent. For Eberle, this property seemed insufficient reason to place hectic fever in the category of remittent fever. A few features of the clinical course could not provide criteria for sound classification.

In the actual practice of medicine, remittent fever became an extremely popular diagnostic term. Some helpful statistics list, year by year, the causes of death in Philadelphia, for the decade of 1831–40. For the year 1831, the date of Eberle's text, 15 deaths were attributed to intermittent fever, 98 to remittent fever, and 92 to typhus. For the decade as a whole, the three categories aggregated 73, 689, and 996, respectively. Typhus included typhoid fever, which did not yet have a separate listing. Clearly, the diagnosis of remittent fever was much more frequent than that of intermittent fever.[4]

As an abstract nosological term, *remittent fever* seemed relatively simple, but in practice it was soon recognized as highly complex and increasingly difficult to define. By the 1840s a strict nosologic schema could no longer provide a reliable conceptual foundation. This becomes clear if we go forward into the 1840s, when further clinical and anatomical studies introduced new data. And with the new data there emerged new conceptual difficulties.

DESCRIPTION OF ANATOMICAL CHANGES

The clinical features of remittent fever and its relation to bilious fever were well recognized by the early 1830s, but the anatomical changes were not described until Thomas Stewardson (1807–78) published his systematic investigations, in 1841 and 1842.[5] He was well versed in the new empiricism, for he had studied in Paris with Louis and had also come under the influence of Gerhard in Philadelphia. His work has a modern ring.

The first paper, of 1841, described the general and pathological aspects. In Philadelphia, remittent fever occurred almost exclusively in July, August, and September. In the three summer months of 1838, the medical wards of the Pennsylvania Hospital received 109 patients, of whom 20 were diagnosed as having remittent fever. Three died; autopsies were performed on two. Stewardson, in charge of the service, based his pathological report on these two, plus five other autopsies on remittent fever patients who died in the following two years.

In all cases, jaundice was a major finding, both clinically and anatomically. The principal morphologic changes affected the liver, which was normal in size or slightly enlarged, but flabby and markedly altered in color and architectural markings. The color was usually described as dull bronze, or a mixture of bronze and olive, with other shades mentioned in different cases. In all instances the spleen was enlarged.

No other pathological finding was constant. Changes in the stomach seemed most worthy of attention, but these findings, together with the enlarged spleens, were also found in other diseases. On the other hand, the change in the liver was "of a character not met with in other diseases," and "it constituted the essential anatomical characteristic of the disease, as it presented itself to our observation."

The anatomical lesions, Stewardson believed, should be considered the result of the disease and not the cause. The cause itself must be sought "in some morbid condition other than what is observed in the solid organs." Investigations on the blood then taking place in France might, he thought, throw some light on this "obscure subject." The solidism that Cullen had supported, with its emphasis on the nervous system, was crumbling, while a new humoralism, attending to changes in the blood, was taking shape.

Stewardson's second paper, of 1842, discussed the clinical aspects and made several important points. He identified three kinds of remittent fever. One he called bilious fever "of a high grade." This fever, relatively rare, might be confused with yellow fever. The second kind he called pernicious, and the third, the "common or ordinary form of the disease."

He tried to distinguish remittent fever from yellow fever but without complete success. Clinical data alone were not enough, and he lamented the lack of adequate anatomical studies that would provide clinicopathological correlations. A study of the "morbid appearances of fever in hot climates . . . conducted by men conversant with pathological anatomy, and considered in connection with the symptoms" would clarify the troublesome points. Such studies could "determine positively the question as to the real distinction between these two diseases [remittent fever and yellow fever], which are still regarded by some as only varieties of one and the same disease." He realized the nature of the problem but lacked the means of solving it.

The pernicious form of remittent fever was known in many parts of the country as congestive fever. Of this he had seen but few cases, and then the inadequate clinical histories did not allow analysis of symptoms. Congestive fever would receive much more detailed attention from other writers of the 1840s.

The third or "ordinary" form of remittent fever comprised most of his cases. In some, when "the remissions are more obscure, and symptoms of the typhoid *state* more or less developed," the distinction between remittent fever and "proper typhoid fever" presented difficulties. When Gerhard, we recall, first studied typhoid fever, he claimed that this disease was quite different from remittent fever. However, further experience showed that clinical differentiation might be quite difficult, and later in the century the composite term *typhomalaria* was widely used to designate the conjunction of symptoms (even if not of diseases).[6]

Stewardson sought the essential nature of remittent fever. Autopsies showed anatomical changes chiefly in the liver, spleen, and stomach. The disease should not be regarded as gastritis, even though gastric "inflammation" seemed more common than in febrile diseases generally. Splenic enlargement was only a consequence and not a cause. The liver was the only organ uniformly affected. The changes here, he said, were certainly not inflammatory. Their essential nature must be sought elsewhere, and he thought the blood was a very probable locus. With his limited tools, Stewardson was nevertheless trying to pinpoint some degree of specificity for remittent fever.

In 1845 John A. Swett (1808–54), working in New York, confirmed Stewardson's findings. Swett presented autopsy data of five fatal cases, all of which showed damage to the liver as the characteristic change. However, he found much less involvement of the stomach than did Stewardson.[7]

PERSISTENT EIGHTEENTH-CENTURY THINKING: JOHN W. MONETTE

Contrasting markedly with the studies in Philadelphia and New York was a long paper by John W. Monette (1803–51), who practiced in Mississippi.[8] Monette studied medicine with his father, in Mississippi, and received the M.D. degree from Transylvania University, in 1825. At that time, the reactionary Charles Caldwell was a leading educational force in Transylvania, and his teachings obviously influenced Monette. The papers of Stewardson and of Monette, when compared, illustrate the differences between nineteenth-century and eighteenth-century thought modes.

For Monette, writing in 1840, fever was a disease of the whole "system." The "exciting cause" (note the singular) was modified by many influences, including age, sex, temperament, climate, season, exposure, and fatigue, "besides other circumstances too tedious to rehearse." These factors "often cause fever to assume the various characteristic forms, which seem to indicate distinct and opposite diseases." He was expressing the familiar concept, that one disease, fever, takes many forms, so varied that they might appear as different diseases. He was denying specificity.

Monette's chief concern lay not with theories but with therapeutics—the practical aspects of medicine. From the standpoint of "pathology," he said, there might be some propriety in distinguishing continued, intermittent, and remittent fevers, but from a therapeutic viewpoint "the distinction is inadmissible." The different forms "so often pass alternately into each other, that the common [i.e., the usual] diagnostic appellation is insufficient to satisfy therapeutic accuracy."

The remittents, with numerous varieties, comprised the great majority of diseases in the South. The particular symptoms depended on the constitution of the patient and on local factors. If the patient had an "irritable constitution," then the disease would "fall upon" the liver or the brain and produce symptoms there. If, however, the patient had a "relaxed and leucophlegmatic temperament," the inciting cause would settle on the alimentary tract, and "profuse watery discharges will ensue." In a plethoric female, however, menorrhagia might result.

Verbal juggling replaced concrete data. In different cases "different groups of organs [were] drawn into the disordered action," and the apparent diversity of diseases represents only the different modes "in which disordered action makes itself cognizable to our senses." Monette had no hopes of a better understanding, which, he thought, "is, and will remain beyond the ken of human research" (p. 94).

VIRULENT CONGESTIVE FEVER: JAMES PARRY'S DESCRIPTIONS

Thomas Stewardson and John Swett described one aspect of remittent fever, affecting the liver. Of the other forms distinguishable on clinical grounds, congestive fever was the most important for both theory and practice. Monette did recognize different kinds of remittent fever. In one group of "sudden and violent cases, properly called *congestive*, there is a collapse of the circulation similar to that in cholera maligna." This he attributed to collapse in the nervous system.

As a diagnosis, congestive fever had a wide currency but without any sharp delineation. In its popular sense, this condition was regarded as part of the "cold stage" that supposedly occurred in every fever. If the usual "reaction" did not follow this initial cold stage, then congestion would occur. According to Cullen, the cold stage represented a vascular phenomenon wherein the blood was forced from the periphery to the internal organs. Ordinarily, a further vascular reaction would return the blood to the surface and bring about the hot stage, with its increase in skin temperature. This centrifugal reaction would automatically eliminate the internal congestion.

If for any reason the blood was not returned to the surface, it remained in the internal organs to constitute a congestion. The surface temperature remained below normal, and autopsies showed a pooling of blood in the viscera. Clinically, the patient would have a cool skin, a pale countenance, a small rapid pulse, and a sense of faintness, oppression, and anxiety.[9] In ordinary intermittent fever, these features did not necessarily indicate a malignant course.

When the diagnosis of remittent fever became prevalent, some remarkable vascular phenomena attracted wide attention. In 1843 Charles Parry (1814?–61?), of Indianapolis, published a highly influential paper in which he described remittent fever as observed in central Indiana.[10] Although the disease ordinarily lasted six to nine days, the patient might die after the second or third paroxysm, two or three days following the onset. Moreover, if the usual treatment for bilious fevers was followed, three-quarters of the patients would die. The cause of death seemed to be "a cessation of the circulation," which we today would call circulatory collapse.

The first paroxysm might follow the usual course and not attract special attention. The second or third paroxysm, however, might be extremely severe, not so much in the actual "rigor" as in the coldness and "death-like hue." There was almost incessant vomiting and purging, often mixed with blood. The discharges did not resemble those of cholera ("rice-water stools") but had "more the appearance of water in which a large portion of recently killed beef has been washed." Sometimes large amounts of blood were passed by rectum.

Thirst was intense. Patients cried out for cold drinks. One patient declared, " 'If I could only have a stream of cold water running through me.' " Respirations sometimes took the form of a deep "double sigh," with long intervals between the end of expiration and the beginning of the next inspiration. The pulse might rise to 120 to 150 per minute, sometimes irregular and with skipped beats.

The capillary circulation seemed "stagnated." The surface of the skin was livid and cold, and often covered with a "cold, clammy, sticky sweat." The skin of the hands was shrivelled and wilted as if they had been "soaked in ley [sic], like a washerwoman's hands." Restlessness was extreme, and patients had a great desire "to get cold air"—what we today would call air hunger. A Hippocratic facies might supervene, the pulse grow more irregular and fluttering, and death take place "easily, as if without cause." Present-day clinicians have completely ignored his superb description of shock.

Parry regarded all this as a disturbance in cardiovascular physiology, but he had no way of reaching a detailed understanding. To treat such desperately ill patients, Parry wanted to "produce reaction" in the circulation. For this he used "stimulating frictions to the hands, arms, and legs, such as cayenne pepper stewed in brandy." He also tried to relieve local internal congestion by cupping or mustard plasters, to bring the blood back from the viscera to the surface. A successful "reaction" might lead to recovery. The pulse might get stronger and more full, the surface grow warmer, the skin become dry, and heat gradually diffuse over the body. When "reaction" had been established, quinine seemed to have great value in preventing recurrence of the paroxysms.

THE QUESTION OF SPECIFICITY

Several other studies followed Parry's report. In 1844, R. G. Wharton, of Mississippi, discussed the disease as it appeared there and in Louisiana.[11] For about a dozen years, he said, congestive fever had been a common condition, recognized by planters as well as physicians. At first it had proved almost uniformly fatal, but more recently the mortality had fallen to only 6 or 8 percent.

Indirectly, Wharton raised the question of specificity. He questioned whether the symptoms of congestive fever were an integral part of remittent fever, such as might define a distinct species. On the other hand, perhaps the symptoms were a sort of symptom complex, with no necessary connection to a particular disease pattern.

Wharton did not phrase the questions in this manner, but he did give an unequivocal answer. Congestive fever, he declared, could "supervene" in every disease of the summer, including intermittents, remittents, continued fever, gastritis and gastroenteritis, and even epidemic influenza. If Benjamin Rush had been aware of the condition, he might have called it a "congestive state."

There was no constant mode of onset, but at some point ominous symptoms might arise. Wharton's clinical descriptions tallied closely with those of Parry, emphasizing oppression, cold extremities, sticky cold perspiration, rapid feeble pulse, sighing respiration, air hunger, and intense thirst. Death, if it occurred, took place within twenty-four to sixty hours from onset.

Physicians were puzzled about the "pathology," by which was meant not the findings of morbid anatomy but the theoretical or conceptual aspects—the "cause" responsible for the condition. The basic defect, according to Wharton, was the weakened state of the heart and arteries, with torpor of the capillaries. This torpor did not result from a "debility" of the heart action. Indeed, the exactly opposite view, that the capillary torpor caused the "oppressed" heart action, seemed "more consistent with sound pathology."

Wharton objected to the name *congestive fever* as "manifestly inappropriate." The disease showed none of the characteristics of fever, and the use of that term might "convey incorrect ideas" in regard to treatment. The therapy he recommended reflected his views of the pathology. The physician must restore circulation. Surface stimulants, like turpentine and capsicum as well as mustard plasters, would help to overcome the torpor of the capillaries. Quinine, which he regarded as a stimulant, could be given in large doses. Thirst he treated with capsicum, which, he believed, gave a centrifugal direction to the blood and thus would relieve the internal congestion. Warmth applied to the extremities was highly recommended. He rejected the use of bloodletting, which would only weaken the heart action still more. His recommended treatment would not have been appropriate for fevers or inflammatory conditions.

In condemning the term *congestive fever,* Wharton declared, "the simple term congestion is much more in accordance with sound pathological, as well as therapeutical principles." In retrospect, we see that he wanted to separate the pattern that had been called congestive fever from the pattern of true fever.

DENIAL OF CONGESTIVE FEVER AS A DISEASE

Both Parry and Wharton admirably described the clinical aspects of congestive fever, but Wharton denied that it was really a fever. Isaac Parrish (1811–52) went one step further and rejected the concept of congestion itself. In 1845 he declared that that term, and the implications behind it, were "not expressive of the true pathology" and therefore could lead to serious errors in practice.[12] Parrish referred to the condition as an "assemblage of symptoms," that is, a pattern that occurred in "a miasmatic district." The same changes were observed in remittent fever, he said, and also occurred in the malignant or pernicious form of intermittent fever.

Parrish objected to the term *congestive fever* on practical as well as theoretical grounds. He declared that many practitioners, when treating a patient, attended to a diagnostic name "without investigating its true meaning" or examining the phenomena that the name supposedly represented. The term *congestion* indicated an "overloaded or turgid state of a particular organ or organs," and furthermore implied that the resulting phenomena "are produced by this fullness." There was no good evidence, he emphasized, that the observed symptoms had actually resulted from congestion of the vital organs. To stress this point, he examined individual symptoms and showed that these occurred in conditions that were definitely not congestive in nature.

Severe thirst, incessant and uncontrollable, was a prime example. It also occurred in uterine hemorrhage when the patient was cold and pulseless from loss of blood; and after surgical procedures, where the operation had resulted in extensive blood loss. Intense thirst indicated a "prostrate condition of the system, and has no relation whatever to congestion of the internal organs."

Similar arguments applied to respiratory distress. The labored respiration in congestive fever resembled the breathing noted in syncope, when no congestion existed in the lungs. The irregular and sighing character was also observed in conditions where the "system" was prostrate from severe hemorrhage. Parrish cited the case of a young woman with a protracted uterine hemorrhage. She died from exhaustion, even while she was demanding that the windows be opened. At autopsy the lungs, instead of being engorged, were unusually pale and bloodless. Furthermore, he noted, a cold and clammy skin occurred after hemorrhages and accidents.

Bloody diarrhea was hard to explain. Supposedly, this feature resulted from engorgement of the intestinal mucosa, but no one had ever demonstrated any remarkable congestion. The asserted relationship was only hypothetical. For Parrish, a more probable explanation lay in the state of the blood or "the relaxed condition of the tissues through which it passes," a view consistent with modern views of increased permeability. These concepts, he noted, although purely hypothetical, seemed preferable to an alleged but unproven congestion.

Parrish further emphasized the advances in the new humoral pathology, emanating chiefly from France, together with the "new lights afforded by animal chemistry." The older solidist doctrine, he believed, probably retarded rather than promoted medical progress. These new concepts, emphasizing the fluids, he regarded "as an auspicious era in the science of medicine."

Further conjectures dealt with what we now call germ theory, but which at that time was rudimentary, indeed. (This aspect I will discuss in the next chapter.) Parrish pointed to changes in the blood that attended "epidemic influences in the atmosphere." For example, if erysipelas was prevalent, a simple wound might result not in ordinary "adhesive inflammation" but rather in a destructive process that might spread and kill the patient. A simple incision in venesection could lead to erysipelas and gangrene. To explain these phenomena, he suggested that they might derive from an "alteration in the properties of the blood." The bloody discharges in so-called congestive fever were also observed in severe injuries and perhaps resulted from "similar alteration in the blood."

Symptoms such as delirium or coma had been confidently attributed to congestion of the brain. However, he pointed out, coma, delirium, and convulsions could occur in two opposite conditions—from too much blood in the brain but also from too little. Lack of blood could produce convulsions and also delirium. These symptoms would not necessarily arise from congestion but might occur in severe blood loss. Moreover, bloody discharges "may be fairly attributed to alterations in the blood itself, combined with laxity of fibre."

Parrish also drew support from therapeutic considerations. If congestion were the real cause of the symptoms, a "depletory practice" should be the only successful method of treatment. But the most experienced physicians condemned depletion as dangerous. Even ordinary intermittent or remittent fevers might be thrown into the dangerous congestive fever by "copious depletion." Indeed, bloodletting, strong catharsis, or severe emesis resulted in a worsened clinical condition.

While Parrish wanted to eliminate the word *congestive,* neither *malignant* nor *pernicious* was a quite satisfactory substitute. He recommended *adynamic,* to indicate the "want of power in the heart and blood vessels" that resulted from the "depressing influence of the malarial poison on the nervous centers." He believed "that a new era is dawning upon medical science" that would help provide answers. More knowledge was needed on the composition and vital properties of the fluids. He was thus supporting the new spirit in medicine and the potential value of physiology and chemistry in solving clinical problems.

Other writers also expressed a dissatisfaction with the concept of congestive fever. As early as 1839, Jacob Bigelow and Oliver Wendell Holmes questioned the validity of the term *congestive fever.*[13] Although blood "preternaturally accumulated" in some of the internal organs, this finding was observed in several distinct diseases. *Congestive fever* was no more specific a term than *delirious fever.* It could not be considered "a distinct disease."

In 1845 a writer in Memphis, Tennessee, declared, "The most intelligent physicians here as well as elsewhere, regard the word *congestive* as indicating no distinct disease, but merely expressive of a *symptom* or *condition* which may be connected with any of the forms of fever."[14] In the same year, a leading South Carolina physician, Samuel Dickson (1798–1892), offered the same message. In published lectures, he too rejected the idea that congestive fever denoted "a separate and distinct type of fever."[15] The proper use demanded an adjectival sense, indicating "certain contingencies which modify the course and symptoms . . . of most types of fever."

In 1848 another southern practitioner, from Alabama, reinforced this general message.[16] He emphasized depression of the "vital force" as a result of a miasmatic poison. He denied that congestive fever was a disease sui generis.

CONGESTIVE FEVER AS VASCULAR COLLAPSE

The alarming symptoms of congestive fever, so admirably described, we today recognize as severe shock. The milder manifestations had seemed little more than the prolongation of the "cold stage" of fever that Cullen had described, sometimes called the "algid" form. The severe form, however, was so striking that it seemed like a separate disease. Nevertheless, thoughtful physicians agreed that it represented only a symptom or manifestation, not a disease entity.

The symptom (or state) might appear in diseases other than fevers—for example, in severe hemorrhage or massive trauma. Modern physiology separates hypovolemic shock, dependent on markedly reduced volume of circulating fluids, from toxic shock, due to the direct action of a poisonous substance. This distinction developed only rather late in the twentieth century, and, of course, was entirely unknown in the midnineteenth century. At that time, the phenomena were explained by such a vague concept as depression of the nervous system. This, in turn, supposedly affected, somehow, the circulatory system.

Although the severe symptoms, which we recognize as shock, produced a great stir during the 1840s, interest in the subject gradually waned. In 1855 Dickson distinguished four clinical types of congestive fever. The condition generally seemed to result from poisoning of the blood through malarious intoxication. But the congestions also "occur and prove fatal when no malarious influences are present." Whatever the cause, he attributed the reaction to a paralysis of the capillary vessels, with suspension of function.[17]

In a textbook of 1858, George B. Wood (1797–1879) devoted a chapter to "Pernicious fever," which included congestive fever. Wood, too, insisted that congestive fever was not a separate disease but that the term should be applied wherever "there is great and sudden prostration and depravation [sic] of the nervous power."[18] This might happen "in all cases of violent shock upon the nervous system." Mere congestion, which was venous, was not the source of the danger, but instead the danger lay in the "nervous prostration" that affected the capillaries. "The innervation of the extreme vessels fails. . . . [These vessels then] allow the watery portions of the blood to ooze through them, almost as through dead membrane." Perhaps Wood had cholera in mind when he wrote this.

After the Civil War, interest in congestive fever seemed to diminish still further. In 1873 Austin Flint's highly regarded textbook, in reviewing the periodic fevers, did not mention congestive fever by name. He noted a form of intermittent fever called algid, characterized by reduced temperature, and cold extremities "like that of a cadaver."[19] Sometimes vomiting and purging are prominent, "leading to a state of collapse, like that in epidemic cholera." Flint did not discuss whether the algid form represented a special entity. The designation *algid* remained in the literature, while the term *congestive fever* gradually lapsed.

EXPANDED KNOWLEDGE ABOUT MALARIA

In 1880 Alphonse Laveran reported peculiar bodies in the blood of patients with intermittent fever.[20] This discovery, of what was soon recognized as the plasmodium, aroused great interest. The word *malaria* was changing its meaning. Instead of indicating miasma, the supposed cause of the disease, the word now identified the disease itself, rigorously defined and identified by the presence of the parasite.

In the United States, William Osler was especially active in the study of malaria. The first edition of his textbook (1892) distinguished three types of pernicious malaria, the comatose, the algid, and the hemorrhagic.[21] In his discussion of the algid form, he expressly mentioned the "intense prostration and feebleness out of all proportion to the local symptoms," and said that the patient might die in "profound asthenia." Other texts, such as James Tyson's (1896), also distinguished the comatose and algid types.[22] The latter showed a collapse comparable to cholera.

Present-day texts show a marked change. In the fourteenth (1975) edition of the *Textbook of Medicine,* the editors devoted only one paragraph to the more severe clinical manifestations in falciparum infections.[23] What had once been called congestive fever received but a single sentence: "Patients may present with signs and symptoms of vascular collapse—so-called algid malaria." By 1985, however, under new editorship, even this sentence disappeared. Anemia, renal failure, cerebral disturbances, and pulmonary edema are mentioned, but algid malaria vanished from this major medical text.[24]

More specialized texts, while mentioning the condition, did not provide much illumination. *Manson's Tropical Diseases* (1982) noted hypothermia, drop in blood pressure, and death in a few hours.[25] Algid malaria allegedly resulted from "overwhelming infection, with collapse, and peripheral vascular failure, probably the result of acute renal failure." Another tropical medicine text, of 1984, gave a somewhat different account.[26] After noting the clinical features that characterized shock, the author declared, "Algid malaria develops during an apparently mild attack of falciparum malaria. Its onset is independent of the prevailing degree of parasitemia or anaemia." The untreated condition was fatal, and the patient died from "vascular failure."

MODERN CONCEPTS OF SHOCK

Present-day concepts of shock distinguish the hypovolemic, septic, and cardiogenic forms, each with its own physiological mechanisms. In congestive fever as described in the 1840s, hypovolemia, from loss of fluids, probably played a part, for the condition was more severe in hot weather and was definitely made worse by a depleting regime. But hypovolemia was probably not the initial or even the main factor. We can, I believe, invoke the broad category of septic (or toxic) shock, related to what earlier writers apparently had in mind when they spoke of "poison."

Richard Root and Merle Sande listed various agents recognized as able to induce septic shock.[27] Besides bacteria, both gram-positive and gram-negative, the authors listed spirochetes, rickettsias, and certain viral and parasitic agents. In the latter group they included toxoplasmas, pneumocystis, and trypanosomes, but did not mention plasmodium. I suggest that plasmodium falciparum should be included in that list. Direct evidence is lacking, but we can rely on analogy to, say, the cholera vibrio and certain gram-negative bacilli. These produce clinical phenomena regarded as toxic shock and resembling those described in the 1840s.

We can only speculate on the reasons why the dramatically intense cases described in the mid-nineteenth century have virtually disappeared. Advances in diagnosis, treatment, and public health measures probably all played a role. Perhaps there were some special strains of the plasmodium that disappeared. At the present moment, the whole subject seems to be "of historical interest only," a concern to which clinicians, immunologists, or pathologists are generally indifferent. For students of intellectual history, however, that interest is profound.

Congestive fever as described in the literature was a recognizable condition. Was it also a condition sui generis in the sense of Nathan Smith? Earlier authors, who gave it a separate place in the classification of fevers, vaguely implied that it was; yet later writers declared that congestive fever was neither fever nor congestion and, indeed, was not a disease at all. What, then, was it? How did it relate to the views of Benjamin Rush, who, rejecting nosology, had insisted on "states" rather than diseases?

In smallpox, clinical appearances were so striking and the course so regular that physicians recognized it as a discrete disease as early as the tenth century. The original recognition derived from clinical observation alone, that is, study of the patient at the bedside. With the fever that William Cullen called typhus, whose differentiation we studied in chapters 4 and 5, the situation was rather different. Clinical appearances were not really sharply defined. No single compelling clinical pattern had as yet marked out a discrete entity.

The views of Rush still preserved great vigor. He insisted that terms like *typhus* or *synochus* had only an adjectival force, indicating properties or states that could appear in various contexts. The occurrence of one state need not have any necessary connection (i.e., inner essential relationship) with other manifestations of disease. He briefly enumerated different states, such as typhus, syno-chal, typhoid, and many others, and described their distinguishing features. For example, the typhus state of fever showed "a weak and frequent pulse, a disposition to sleep, a torpor of the alimentary canal, tremors of the hands." His descriptions called attention to the symptoms the patient was immediately manifesting, without regard for any unifying temporal course.

Physicians who rejected the authority of Rush nevertheless continued to use terms like *typhoid* (or even *typhus*) in an adjecti-val sense, to describe symptoms found in varied conditions. These terms, when used as adjectives, referred to a symptom or state not at all self-subsistent.

Wood admirably clarified this distinction. He stressed the differ-ence between nonspecific properties, symptoms, or states that oc-curred in many different diseases and an entity that was specific, or sui generis. He pointed to a "peculiar febrile disease, distinct from all others, characterized by a peculiar group of symptoms, and produced probably by a peculiar cause, to which the name *typhus* or *typhus fever*, is attached."[28] The word *peculiar*, repeated several times, corresponds to our presentday term *specific*.

However, he continued, in other febrile diseases, features "iden-tical or closely analogous" with those that characterized typhus were frequently found. When this occurred "the epithet *typhous* or *typhoid* is applied. . . . Thus, we speak of a typhous or typhoid condition of bilious fever, yellow fever, small pox, measles, pneumo-nia, dysentery, &c.; or, with greater brevity, of *typhous pneumonia*, *typhous dysentery*, &c." He went on, "This distinction between the peculiar disease named typhus fever, and the analogous state of system met with in other diseases, indicated by the adjective epi-thets typhous and typhoid" must be constantly kept in mind "in order to avoid serious error" (ibid.).

Thus, in 1858 Wood seemed to reaffirm Rush's views in a more limited context. Wood objected strongly to the name *typhoid fever* that Louis had fastened on the medical world. Many different terms had already been applied to that entity, such as typhus mitior, nervous fever, dothinenteritis, follicular enteritis, enteromesenteric fever, and the like. Wood himself proposed the simple term *enteric fever*.

Louis's designation, *typhoid fever*, Wood considered thoroughly bad. In the first place, the disease was not "essentially typhoid," that is, it did not necessarily show the stuporous qualities implied by the adjective typhoid. Furthermore, many other febrile conditions might equally assume the "typhoid form." Bilious fever, yellow fever, plague, the exanthemata, and various fevers secondary to inflammation (phlegmasias) could also show typhoid symptoms, although admittedly not so frequently. Diseases whose manifestations might in part resemble those found in typhus would not, merely for that reason, be called typhus. In Wood's terms, many different diseases might "become typhoid" (pp. 337–38).

THE DISEASE ENTITY: ITS RELATION TO PATTERN AND SYMPTOM COMPLEX

The problems that Wood discussed center upon the concept of pattern. By *pattern,* I mean an aggregate of phenomena that cohere, not by mere chance, but by some inner connection. There was a "belonging together," through some internal nonrandom relationship that extended over a period of time. For a better understanding, we may compare the three diseases or conditions, smallpox, typhoid fever, and congestive fever, as representing patterns.

A typhoid state, for example, combined certain features affecting the pulse, the mental condition, bodily strength, and other physiological processes. These indicated a definite but limited clinical togetherness, a pattern of a sort, since the different features hung together as if through some inner connection. The typhoid state, however, was regarded as a symptom and not a disease. How, then, does a pattern called a symptom differ from a pattern called a disease?

The answer seems clear. A symptom, itself a small pattern, is only one component of a larger pattern, whose complexity can render it unique. The distinction between a symptom pattern and a disease pattern is readily illustrated by an analogy from architecture. If we look at a pediment, or a frieze, or a Doric column, we find that each shows certain features arranged in a describable pattern. Pediments, friezes, and columns are widely distributed in various buildings, of which they are components. When, however, these component features are combined with other elements into a larger and complex pattern, we get a class of buildings, represented by, say, the Parthenon.

A clear distinction existed between a symptom and a disease. A symptom was a subordinate pattern, in itself nonspecific, that could participate in many other and larger patterns that represented diseases.

These concepts were applicable to congestive fever. By the 1850s there was general agreement that congestive fever, with all its dramatic phenomena, should not be considered a disease sui generis. Parrish, as we have seen, called it "an assemblage of symptoms," a view that William Tuck echoed with the phrase "symptom or condition." The same symptoms might appear in other diseases that showed quite different manifestations, such as intermittent fever, remittent fever, cholera, hemorrhage, and trauma, among others.

Elisha Bartlett, when discussing congestive fever, recognized that a coherent group of clinical findings might occur in widely distinct diseases. The prefix *congestive,* he said, expressed "a pathologic state or condition, which may exist in different diseases."[29] The parallelism between the adjective *typhoid* (used chiefly in the continued fevers) and the adjective *congestive* (noted especially in the periodic fevers) is noteworthy. In *a* congestive fever, as in *a* typhoid fever, the adjectival sense denotes a property that may occur in many quite diverse conditions.

The so-called congestive fever would then be a rather complex symptom or state. Symptom, state, or condition were used quite interchangeably. In present-day usage the term *symptom complex* provides a way to distinguish symptoms from diseases and specific diseases from the nonspecific.

Symptom complex is not as formidable a term as it might sound. Let me give a simple example. If for any reason a loop of small bowel becomes kinked and does not shake itself loose, the bowel can become obstructed, producing what is technically known as ileus. When I was a medical student, I learned a simple mnemonic that, like so many trivia, remains in the memory after more weighty concepts have disappeared:

Ileus is a symptom complex, known throughout creation
Tympanites, vomiting, pain, and obstipation

Each of these terms represents a symptom that, by itself, might appear in a great variety of separate conditions. When, however, the symptoms appear concurrently, they form a pattern that characterizes ileus and permits a ready diagnosis.

Medical students are pleased when they see how clearly each of these symptoms can be traced to the underlying mechanical obstruction. They become troubled, however, when they learn that the same symptoms can occur without mechanical obstruction. For reasons not clearly understood, there may be a failure of innervation, and the normal movement of the bowel may be paralyzed. In such an instance, physicians speak of paralytic ileus, in contrast to obstructive ileus. Sometimes the clinical differentiation may be difficult.

If we call ileus a symptom, we do not distinguish it from its component features, each of which is also a symptom. However, to call ileus a symptom complex indicates an aggregate or pattern of components, each of which would be a symptom simpliciter.

We cannot call ileus a specific disease, comparable to smallpox. The latter has not only its characteristic pattern of symptoms but also a definite and specific cause. John Armstrong, we recall, emphasized this point early in the century and postulated as cause a specific contagion (which eventually passed from the stage of postulation to an empirical demonstration). To make a simple and effective discrimination, we may call smallpox a disease and ileus a symptom complex. Both are patterns, but these patterns differ profoundly.

As originally described in the literature, congestive fever should be called shock. I suggest a certain parallel between ileus and shock. Both could appropriately be called symptom complexes that may result from many causes. Armstrong would have called them nonspecific.

We have already noted the growing realization that causation had an important role in identifying a specific disease entity. This realization marks a significant step in the transformation of thought modes. As the basis for classification, Boissier de Sauvages, in the eighteenth century, rejected etiology in favor of clinical symptoms. In the nineteenth century, etiology became an essential feature in the identification of disease entities.

So far in the discussion I have used the word *cause* in a rather simplistic sense. Indeed, the medical usage of the term may seem rather naive and inconsistent. However, as the discipline of bacteriology developed, new meanings became attached to the notion of cause. In the next chapter I will take up some of these changes and the way they relate to the agents in the realm of microbiology.

7

Germ Theory,
Causation, and
Specificity

T HE TERM *GERM THEORY* IS EASY TO USE AND HARD
to define. Hence I will merely indicate in broad strokes the
meaning it has here, namely, a vague mass of data and concepts
having to do with the causes of infectious disease, especially the
febrile diseases. While some of the component ideas can be traced
back to antiquity and much more to the sixteenth, seventeenth,
and eighteenth centuries, the greatest development occurred in
the last quarter of the nineteenth century, with the so-called golden
age of bacteriology. Despite the long lineage, this aggregate of ideas
exerted no effect on Benjamin Rush but profoundly influenced
William Osler. I deal essentially, then, with a nineteenth-century
phenomenon.

Any approach through the traditional history of bacteriology,
would traverse a field already well cultivated in both scholarly and
popular literature.[1] I want, rather, to explore the way the concepts
and data inherent in germ theory took root in medicine and over-
came substantial inertia. It is not enough to point to this or that
discovery in bacteriology as a step in medical progress. New data
acquired significance only when the mental set, or intellectual
framework, became receptive. There was a mutual interplay, so
that new modes of thinking provided a favorable environment for
new ideas, and at the same time the new ideas helped to alter the
intellectual framework. Consequently, we must study the slow
modification in medical thinking resulting from new insights.

This approach gives primacy to the twin concepts of causation and specificity, together with their interrelation. The age-old search to identify the causes of disease led to increasing discrimination, and this, in turn, eventually involved the idea of specificity. The search for causes took place within a conceptual framework that changed gradually but continuously and reached a high point when specific bacteria were accepted as having a unique relationship to particular diseases.

GREATER PRECISION REGARDING CAUSATION

In this chapter I will trace some steps whereby physicians expanded their ideas of causation and specificity, so that by the last quarter of the nineteenth century a virtual medical revolution had taken place. In this presentation, when I speak of disease I am referring chiefly to the febrile diseases, and more particularly the essential fevers—the *febres* of William Cullen—together with the exanthemata, which served as a model.

I start with the framework of causation generally accepted in the early part of the eighteenth century, with its own nomenclature. A disease was an effect, the factors that led up to it were the causes. For understanding a disease, a multiplicity of causal factors was recognized, separated into various categories.

The nineteenth-century division into proximal and remote causes originally depended on their temporal closeness to the effect. By 1840, however, the notion of a separate proximal cause was being generally abandoned. It was recognized as not a true cause but only an alternative description of the disease process, couched in physiological terms. With this change in attitude, the concept of proximal cause disappeared, and the burden of explanation fell on the remote causes. These embraced any factor that influenced the disease, regardless of temporal proximity. Some of these remote factors might have acted for a long time, others only briefly. They differed among themselves not only in temporal relevance but also in importance and constancy. Furthermore, they differed in their locus of action. Some, like the weather or the physical surroundings, composed part of the external environment; other factors, like the "temperaments," were part of the body and helped to determine the way the body reacted to the environment.

There developed a more logical separation of remote causes

into two types, predisposing and exciting. For example, of many individuals who might be exposed to the same weather conditions, some would get sick, others would remain well. An environmental factor that could induce disease (i.e., an exciting cause) thus encountered different kinds of reactivity. Whatever features determined the way the individual would react constituted the predisposing causes. And whatever induced a reaction would be an exciting cause. These terms, already current but rather vague in the seventeenth and eighteenth centuries, became increasingly precise in the nineteenth century. The study of infectious diseases, eventuating in the discovery of bacterial agents, exemplifies very well the whole trend toward greater precision.

CONTAGION AS A REMOTE CAUSE

Preliminary to the survey, I mention the problem, intrusive in the eighteenth century, whether a given disease was contagious or infectious. Today the terms are synonymous, and present-day medical students wonder how the one might differ from the other. In the early nineteenth century, however, the distinction was significant, and its loss illustrates the increasing precision of that era in regard to causation.

A contagious disease spread by contact with a sick person. The actual transmission took place through a material agent, a contagion, that passed from the patient to someone else through direct or indirect contact. In contrast is the term *infection,* which derives from the Latin *inficere,* to tinge, dye, or stain.[2] If the ambient air contained the disease agent or exciting cause, it could affect a healthy person at any time, regardless of any actual contact with someone already ill. The classic example, frequently mentioned in earlier chapters, was intermittent fever, whose exciting cause was considered to be malaria, or miasma, or tainted air. There was no other mode of spread, for in intermittent fever even the most intimate contact would not transmit the disease.

From the practical standpoint, the question whether disease did or did not spread by contact had obvious importance for public health measures and social behavior. This becomes clear in historical reactions to epidemics such as yellow fever, cholera, and poliomyelitis. Today we have similar concern with the autoimmune deficiency syndrome (AIDS).[3] Yet the mode of spread was only one property among many, and with further study a distinction between a contagious and an infectious spread seemed not very important. Attention focused rather on the properties of the responsible agent, or exciting cause.

THE OLDER TRADITION: JOHN ARMSTRONG

John Armstrong expressed the above distinction clearly. An atmosphere, he said, was infected "when it excites fever in those who are exposed to it without communicating an attribute to the fever by which it can propagate its kind indefinitely." At issue was the multiplication of the actual agent. Without such multiplication, the agent would not pass from one person to another. A contagion, in contrast, was "capable of maintaining itself by successive re-productions in those upon whom it operates."[4] A contagion could pass serially from one person to another. The actual quantity of this agent might initially have been exceedingly minute, yet within the body it multiplied to an enormous degree, always maintaining the same properties and always inducing the same disease in others. Armstrong believed "that a fever is never contagious except it originates from a *specific* cause" (ibid., p. 266). The concept of specificity was becoming increasingly important.

While a contagion could be regarded as a specific agent capable of multiplication and serial transmission, the status of so-called infectious fevers was not so distinct. As we saw in chapter 4, Armstrong offered a solution when he classified fevers according to two principles. A fever could be contagious or noncontagious; it could also be specific or nonspecific. Contagious fevers he placed in a single group he called typhus. Of the noncontagious fevers, the intermittents (or agues) resulted from a specific causative agent in the atmosphere that derived from decomposition of vegetation under conditions of heat and moisture. Although this agent (which we now recognize as the mosquito) could not multiply within the body as a contagion did, he regarded it as nevertheless specific.

There remained a large group of noncontagious febrile conditions that were attributed to a variety of other factors. That whole group Armstrong designated "common continued fevers." They might proceed from many quite different causes and therefore were nonspecific as well as noncontagious.

The focus of interest was changing. Whether a fever was contagious or infectious seemed much less important than whether it was specific or nonspecific. This problem, in turn, entailed other difficulties. Could a disease, originally nonspecific, become specific? How did disease agents arise? What were the relationships of general and specific causes, and what did these terms really mean?

Physicians devoted increasing attention to studying the properties or agents and their relationships to fevers. According to prevalent theory, in intermittent fevers the morbific agent arose from the action of heat and moisture on decaying vegetable matter, as found in swamps and marshes. Perhaps an analogous process could explain some of the problems in regard to typhus (referring to the rickettsial form).

Typhus was a cold-weather disease, appearing under conditions of overcrowding, with close physical contact, poverty, and poor hygiene. Normal secretions accumulated and underwent decay. Sometimes the disease was highly contagious and appeared in epidemic form, but at other times it seemed only slightly contagious. Cullen had vaguely suggested that the morbific agent, whatever it might be, came into being when certain environmental factors acted on the secretions of the patient. He pointed out that "effluvia" were constantly arising from the living human body. If these secretions were not diffused in the atmosphere, they could, under certain conditions, "acquire a singular virulence." They could then transform into a contagious agent.[5]

Typhus seemed definitely related to poverty, overcrowding, and filth. Through heat, moisture, and lack of ventilation, Cullen believed, bodily secretions, which normally dissipated into the air, might become virulent. This new virulent property could then, through contact with another person, induce a specific and transmissible disease.

Cullen was drawing a rough analogy with intermittent fever. The common denominator was an effluvium, which in the one case arose from a marsh or swamp, in the other, from the human body. In either case, under certain circumstances, an effluvium could become transformed into a disease-producing agent, regardless of whether the origin was vegetable or animal. With this analogy in mind, Cullen wanted to designate the agents of disease as "*Human or Marsh Effluvia*," (ibid., par. 85), rather than as contagion or miasma. The role of the atmosphere, so important with intermittent fevers, was thus being extended to contagious diseases such as typhus.

A BROADER VIEW OF CONTAGION: JOHN EBERLE

Cullen's views, stated somewhat tentatively, were expanded and codified in the next half century or so, especially by the American physician John Eberle. Eberle's views on causation, published in the 1830s, provide a baseline for studying the further development of germ theory.[6]

Eberle defined miasma as the class of febrific agents that had a gaseous form and acted through the atmosphere. He distinguished two types of infectious effluvia. One, the common marsh miasma, or malaria, he called koniomiasmata, having the sense of a common origin. He described many of the known properties of that agent.

The second type or variety, the idiomiasmata, were "generated by the decomposition of the matter of perspiration, and the other excretions of the animal body" (ibid., vol. 1, p. 48). The concept seems an ad hoc elaboration to explain the clinical aspects of typhus (the rickettsial form) and to bring this disease into relationship with other forms of fever. Clinical experience with typhus showed that it sometimes remained quite limited to certain areas and sometimes spread widely, as in a severe epidemic.

Eberle followed Cullen: when animal secretions and exhalations accumulated in a limited space and "deteriorate the atmosphere," they might undergo decomposition. There resulted a morbific agent, the idiomiasmata, "that are always quite limited in the sphere of their influence." Typhus was not necessarily a contagious disease, but it might, "under peculiar circumstances, generate a specific virus which is capable of exciting the same disease in others" (p. 50).

The disease typhus did not arise automatically from the effluvium, for the idiomiasmata arising from the human body became innocuous when exposed to abundant fresh air. For an epidemic to arise, the effluvium had to "decompose," and the disease thus generated might then pass from one person to another. Eberle suggested that perhaps the idiomiasmata attached itself (he frequently used the plural noun in a singular construction) to the clothes of individuals or to other substances that permitted transport over long distances. It seemed likely that propagation occurred through "a specific virus, generated by morbid secretion, and conveyed as other contagions of an aeriform character are conveyed." If conveyed by fomites, then the disease "must possess all the characteristics of a veritable contagion" (p. 50). There was as yet no notion of an animal vector. Fomites, as agents of transfer, were inanimate and merely passive.

Two features here call for comment. The mere effluvia of the animal body were not by themselves pathogenic; the disease arose only when there was "decomposition," or putrefaction, of the secretions. The actual morbific agent responsible for typhus would thus have arisen by spontaneous generation. Even when transfer of the disease did occur, Eberle seemed unsure whether the effluvia had impregnated the clothing and allowed a fresh generation of the actual agent to develop de novo or whether the original spontaneous generation had produced a "true contagion," comparable to that of smallpox.

The miasmatic diseases could show marked clinical variations, manifesting themselves as intermittent and remittent fevers, bilious fever, or yellow fever. Eberle explained this by postulating variation in the "powers" of the koniomiasmata. He suggested that the material undergoing decomposition could have different proportions of animal and vegetable substances. Variations in the kind of material might induce "a corresponding diversity in the essential morbific qualities of the miasmata evolved from them." In groping toward specificity, he suggested a quantitative variation in composition, but he also emphasized "a corresponding diversity in the essential morbific *qualities* of the miasmata" (p. 52; emphasis added).

Disease, however, depended not only on the exciting agent but also on the predisposing factors. Different individuals exposed to the same miasmas might contract either an intermittent fever, or a mild remittent fever, or a malignant bilious fever, or a bilious colic, or a dysentery—or they might escape entirely. This diversity Eberle explained by variations in "the physiological state of the animal economy, of idiosyncrasy, of temperament, predisposition, and of accidental external causes" (p. 52).

Eberle was uncertain where the responsibility lay. Sometimes he veered toward a special quality of the exciting cause, other times to peculiarities of the predisposing causes, that is, the peculiarities inherent in the individual. People varied greatly in their "power of resisting injurious influences." The prick of a needle might in one person induce "constitutional irritation," in another, syncope, in another, tetanus, or in another, no harmful effect at all. This, to him, indicated "a natural or *constitutional* predisposition to disease," quite independent of external causal factors. Such a constitutional aptitude to disease would relate, he thought, to "the peculiar organization of the animal system" (p. 29).

Exciting agents also varied in their properties, such as differences in composition and in "potency." Increased potency could induce fevers of more violent grade. Moreover, miasmas could cause numerous other "affections," including dysentery, cholera, diarrhea, plague, and yellow fever. Eberle quoted Joseph Smith—the same Dr. Smith we met in chapter 5—who believed that despite the diversities of circumstances, the "pathology or essential nature is everywhere the same" (p. 54). Eberle refused to accept dogmatic authority. He admitted that Smith's assertion seemed probable but believed the question must be solved not by reasoning "but by close observation and careful experience" in various climates and localities. Eberle himself, however, lacked the training in observation that younger physicians like Gerhard had acquired.

When we read the textbooks of this period we see how physicians were searching for the explanation that the germ theory would ultimately provide. Eberle was not really an original thinker, but he did present the current problems and also the solutions derived from existing knowledge and attitudes. His formulations, however, lacked the key pieces in the puzzle.

EXPANDED INSIGHTS: JACOB BIGELOW AND OLIVER WENDELL HOLMES

By the early 1830s the concept of specificity had made considerable progress. The decline of formal nosology, which had arranged diseases by their symptoms, opened the way for a more dynamic approach. John Armstrong stimulated progress when, stressing etiology, he divided diseases into those with specific and those with nonspecific causes. At the same time, progressive physicians, showing increased powers of discrimination, separated conditions that had seemed surprisingly similar. The identification of typhoid fever as an entity, although it needed two more decades for complete acceptance, emphasized the importance of specificity.

Eberle, as part of the newer trend, may be compared with two other Americans, Jacob Bigelow and Oliver Wendell Holmes, writing a few years later. Bigelow, a progressive and independent thinker, was entirely American trained. Holmes, now more famous as a literary figure than a physician, had received much of his medical training in Paris, and played a major role in introducing the new French ideas and methodology into the United States.

As noted earlier, the two men edited an American edition (1839) of Marshall Hall's British textbook.[7] New material, clearly marked, presented their own views, to replace what Hall had originally written.

In accordance with the current modes of thinking, Bigelow and Holmes separated causes into the general and the specific. A general cause could produce several different diseases, each of which, however, might also arise from other agencies. General causes would also include hereditary tendencies, hygienic influences, and various other external factors, any of which could play a role in many different conditions. In contrast, the "poison" of smallpox, as a specific disease, could produce only smallpox.

General causes might be predisposing or exciting. Predisposing causes, rendering the "system" susceptible to a disease, could be internal or external, that is, inhering in either the individual or the environment. The exciting causes were "all those influences which by their immediate impressions induce any disease" (ibid., p. 68). Even though they used the term *immediate*, Bigelow and Holmes explicitly rejected the old view of "proximate cause." This they regarded as part of the disease and not a cause at all (p. 67n).[8]

The exciting causes, which supposedly precipitated the disease, could not be well circumscribed, for they might include almost any influence acting on the body. If the predisposing causes were sufficiently intense, then a slight stimulus, ordinarily innocuous, might suffice to precipitate a disease. In dealing with general causes, it was often impossible to tell which factors could be called predisposing and which ones precipitating or exciting.

For example, substances introduced into the intestinal tract or into the lungs might act as either predisposing or exciting causes, depending on circumstances. So, too, psychological factors could, as predisposing factors, lay the groundwork for disease, or they could act as precipitating factors. Emotion might bring about apoplexy, and both jaundice and erysipelas "are sometimes brought on by a fit of anger or other excitement of the passions."[9] The attribution of erysipelas to a specific germ was still far in the future.

Bigelow and Holmes then discussed specific causes, referring to a broad spectrum of diseases, both contagious and noncontagious. Noncontagious causes included many substances of mineral origin, such as mercury, lead, copper, and coal, all of which led to specific morbid conditions. So, too, with many gases, such as nitrous oxide, or "exhilarating gas." Correlatively, there were also substances of vegetable origin, including numerous alkaloids, that were considered specific in producing their effects.

Among specific agents of vegetable origin, Bigelow and Holmes placed the atmospheric poison generated by heat and moisture acting on vegetable matter at a certain stage of decomposition. This poison constituted malaria, the miasma responsible for paroxysmal fevers. As a specific agent and also as a product of vegetable origin, it seemed analogous to, say, strychnine. The one was gaseous, the other solid, but both, when introduced into the body, caused a specific disease that was noncontagious. These analogies were not to be ignored. They sharpened the concept of specificity but did not contribute to germ theory.

However, we do approach closer when we examine the specific causes of animal origin (pp. 79–83). These were enumerated under four heads. One was "decomposing animal matter"—putrid flesh. Authorities, however, disagreed regarding the harmful effects these "emanations" might have. Although effluvia might be unpleasant to the senses, they did not necessarily pose the danger to health that popular opinion had believed.

Holmes and Bigelow mentioned two other categories but quickly passed them over. The "venomous secretions" of certain animals, such as snakes, were specific. So too was the interaction between certain forms of flesh and some personal idiosyncrasies. The phraseology, while obscure, clearly related to certain allergic phenomena. Bigelow and Holmes did not pursue the subject, but other writers did discuss these phenomena in greater detail. The text referred to substances of both animal and vegetable origin and noted such phenomena as hay fever, rose fever, and sensitivity to shellfish. All these were noncontagious but specific.

Of special import was the fourth category, comprising "the products of diseased action" and representing the specific contagious diseases. As their first example, the authors pointed to the "malignant pustule"—anthrax—which originated "from the dead bodies of animals in a certain diseased condition." This disease could be transferred by inoculation—it was contagious.

In this connection I would again emphasize that the word *contagion* sometimes meant to Bigelow and Holmes a mode of spread and sometimes the agent by which the spread took place. For some diseases, the contagion (or agent) might be merely one of several possible causes; in other diseases, the only cause. In the former instance, typhus served as the prime example. In "genuine" typhus (the rickettsial form), the disease was generated, somehow, under conditions of overcrowding, poverty, lack of cleanliness, and bad food, which they saw as the principal causal factors. Once the disease was generated, something might happen so that propagation could occur through the atmosphere. A contagion had been produced.

This view, dating back to Cullen more than half a century earlier and already discussed by Eberle, revealed a vast gap between the factors that induced the disease and the contagious principle that transmitted the disease. There was a "process of diseased action," but the nature of that action was entirely unclear. A long period had to elapse before a solution emerged.

CAN GENERAL CAUSES BECOME SPECIFIC CONTAGIOUS PRINCIPLES?

At issue was the concept that a disease could manifest specific contagious properties, even though it arose from factors that were deemed nonspecific. While typhus was a widely accepted example, Bigelow and Holmes called attention to others. They were undecided about the contagious nature of dysentery, which was "commonly produced by other causes" but which still might be contagious. Many other diseases of spontaneous origin could subsequently be propagated by contagion, such as purulent ophthalmia, mumps, tinea capitis, and yaws. Some diseases originating in lower animals, such as hydrophobia, vaccinia, and perhaps glanders, after they had developed in animals, would also be included as contagious and, therefore, specific. Once the contagious principle was developed, it would "reproduce the same series of symptoms and no other." That seemed the essence of contagion.

The transition between a general cause and a specific contagious principle was bridged by vague terms, such as *decomposition* or *corruption of an effluvium,* with indefinite reference to something called *vital action.* So far as concerns germ theory, all this represents a form of spontaneous generation, the development of a specific contagious principle from nonspecific causes. Although spontaneous generation has been admirably discussed in the histories of bacteriology, as a "scientific" controversy settled by experimentation, the histories uniformly ignored that problem in its clinical setting. Nevertheless, this aspect formed a major issue in the medical science of the day.

A different class of contagious disease resulted solely from contact with already infected cases. In this category, the disease arose only "from the intercourse, direct or indirect, with those already affected." With such ailments, the ordinary general causes were not operative. Included were smallpox, scarlatina, measles, and some of the nonfebrile infections such as syphilis and gonorrhea.

Among the contagious fevers, smallpox continued to hold a special position as the model of specificity. There was a clarity about the disease that no other disease (except, perhaps measles) could achieve. Compared to smallpox, other febrile conditions showed many similarities but also many differences. The key to the puzzle seemed to lie in the realm of causation. Physicians were trying to explain the difficulties by making a sharper analysis.

By the early 1840s, new influences were becoming manifest, and the whole intellectual climate seemed to be changing. Fresh clinical observations were proving suggestive, and especially in Europe technical advances opened new conceptual paths. In research centers abroad, experimentation flourished. Physicians posed questions to nature and tried to wrest the answers from experiments. The results, yielding a flood of medical literature, required evaluation and interpretation.

In the United States the experimental approach lagged, but

physicians continued to make sharp clinical observations, to critically examine their own data, and, with some time lapse, to evaluate the newer data coming from Europe.

NEW INFLUENCES: THEORY OF FERMENTS

In the 1830s, major advances were taking place in what would now be called the basic sciences, and while these new advances had no immediate effect on clinical medicine, they did have a profound effect on medical theory. There gradually developed a new intellectual framework within which clinical disease could find new explanations. The advances, for the time being, all took place in Europe, but the new experimental data and their theoretical implications did spread to the United States after a relatively short lag.

Chemists in the early nineteenth century were transforming the science of physiology and, with the new discipline of physiological chemistry ("animal chemistry"), made fundamental contributions to the theories of disease. In regard to infectious diseases, one major approach lay through the study of fermentation and its relation to the action of yeasts. In this field, Justus von Liebig was an outstanding contributor. While fermentation is discussed in histories of bacteriology,[10] a contemporary overview, particularly relevant to medicine, was offered by the British physician Thomas Watson (1792–1862).

I quote from Watson's text, *Lectures on the Principles and Practice of Physic,* which for thirty years was considered "the chief English text-book of medicine."[11] There were five British editions, from 1843 to 1871, and six American editions, from 1844 to 1872. The American text of 1847, which I have used, differed little from the American edition of 1845, which in turn was virtually identical with the British text of 1843. Thus, while the American edition bears the date 1847, the views are really those of several years earlier.

Watson regarded contagion as a kind of poison that acted primarily on the blood. He divided poisons into the inorganic and the organic. The latter, when received into the blood, were capable of multiplication. For the possible mode of action, he tentatively adopted the views of Justus von Liebig. Watson summarized the views of Liebig and their relation to medicine (ibid., pp. 932–34).

According to new chemical theory, if an animal poison was introduced into the body, the reaction in the blood resembled the fermentation resulting from yeast. Yeast is a "putrefying gluten" that had its own "intestine motion." This it could communicate to the elements of sugar contained in the solution and thereby break them down into simpler forms. (*Gluten,* a term cognate to *glue,* had an extremely vague meaning, connected, somehow, with constituents of living creatures, especially the components of an "albuminous" nature.) If the substrate to which the original gluten (or yeast) was added should itself contain a suitable gluten, this could undergo a reaction and become gradually transformed into the yeast substance. In this way, the yeast multiplied and reproduced itself by using the gluten in the containing fluid.

This provided an analogy for infections. The virus of smallpox, well recognized as multiplying in the body, produced changes in the blood, and these permitted the poison to reproduce itself from the constituents of that fluid. Since this process disturbed the workings of the animal economy, the patient manifested disease.

In fermentation, if the solution did not contain any gluten, the reproduction of the yeast did not take place. In human infection, by analogy, if the blood did not contain the suitable gluten, the poisonous agent did not multiply. "In order that a specific animal poison should effect its own reproduction in the blood, and excite that commotion in the system which results from the formation and expansion of the new virus, it is requisite that a certain ingredient (analogous to the gluten in the brewer's sweetwort) should be present in the blood; and this ingredient must have a definite relation to the given poison."

Then, after describing Liebig's "ingenious theory," Watson declared that he did not give it complete credence. The theory did offer a "plausible explanation" of certain facts, such as the origin of the disease from an animal poison and the vast increase of the "specific virus" during the illness. Watson stated, "I entertain the theory, therefore, until a better one is propounded." The theory, he pointed out, has the "incidental merit, that it involves no risk of practical error." He was saying that the theory, whether accepted or not, did not affect therapy.

According to the analogy, for an infectious agent to multiply, the blood had to contain very specific ingredients, lumped together as gluten. If these were not present, multiplication would not take place, and infection would not occur. So too, if the quantity of gluten were exhausted, multiplication would cease. Such a phenomenon would offer one explanation for the recovery of the patient.

EVIDENCE FROM A DISEASE OF SILKWORMS

Liebig's original theory was purely chemical but with modification become related to the animalcular hypothesis.[12] This maintained that diseases were caused by living creatures. Its earliest forms had been propounded solely on theoretical grounds, but with the advent of microscopy, minute creatures were actually visible (Leeuwenhoek's "little animals"). There had been speculation that perhaps these motile particles seen under the microscope might be agents of disease. The whole history of the "contagium animatum" is well presented in Bulloch.[13]

Hypothesis is one thing, firm evidence quite another. In the 1830s some cogent evidence appeared, but the most striking data dealt with animal and not human disease. In 1836 Antonio Bassi (1773–1856) published an epoch-making study of muscardine, a disease of silkworms that threatened the silk industry with ruin.

Bassi was a civil servant and only an amateur scientist, but through intense study and research he proved conclusively the causative role of a specific fungus in a specific infectious disease— a task that no physician had as yet achieved. Again, we can best appreciate his work on muscardine through the eyes of a younger contemporary, Jakob Henle (1809–85). That gifted pathologist, who published his study of miasmas and contagions a few years after Bassi wrote, clearly perceived the significance of the latter's researches.[14]

In the silkworm, the characteristic signs of the disease appeared as a rule only after death, when the body became covered with a white powdery efflorescence shown to be a fungus or mold. In the natural infection, the fungus, when introduced into the body of the worm, grew and killed the animal. Then it "bores through the skin, and a forest of fungi appears, which luxuriates" if the atmosphere was moist and warm. Later "the small cryptogams lose their water, dry up and change to a powder, which contains the germs." These readily disseminated into the air at the slightest movement. They spread widely, remained suspended in the air, and could attach themselves to anything.

Experimentally, the disease could at first be readily transmitted by inoculation from spots inside the body. This material, however, soon became "ineffectual," but then the disease could still be transmitted through vegetations of the surface. The "germs" retained their infectious properties for at least three years.

Bassi believed that only the spores could transmit the disease. Henle, however, referred to other workers who demonstrated that the transmission could also occur through the filamentous processes.

There was a clear distinction between the vegetative or filamentous forms of the fungus and the spores. The latter represented the strict meaning of the term *germ,* that is, the primordium out of which something else arose and the source of the mature entity. This original usage persists when we speak of germinal epithelium in embryology; or metaphorically, of the germ of an idea. Properly speaking, a spore is a germ, the fungus filament is not. Neither is a bacterium. The term *disease germ* represented an extension, referring to that out of which the whole disease pattern ensues. In this sense, the spore would be the disease germ, and by further extension, any pathogenic microorganisms were called germs. And then, by further extension, microorganisms of any type, pathologic or not, were called germs. This usage persists today when popular advertisements for antiseptics boast of the power to "kill germs."

IMPROVED MICROSCOPY AND ITS EFFECTS

A critical element in the developing germ theory was the changing status of microscopy. In the 1820s, technical advance made possible greatly improved lenses with much sharper definition. The improved accuracy eventually led to the concept of cells and to the so-called cell theory enunciated by Schleiden and Schwann. The eventual impact of this theory quite transformed all of pathology and clarified numerous troublesome problems, especially in inflammation and neoplasia.[15]

This aspect, however, I will not take up. For our purposes, special relevance attaches to the persisting limitations of microscopy, despite the technical advances. There was as yet no adequate means of differential staining nor of sectioning soft tissue. (Schleiden and Schwann, when working on their theory, studied cartilage from which reasonably thin sections could quite readily be prepared free hand.) Unstained smears and wet preparations provided the basis for most observations. Under these circumstances, there was extreme difficulty in evaluating the abundant granular material (in contrast to filaments). Spores, fat globules, cellular debris, as well as many bacteria and yeasts, would be difficult to differentiate.

Pathologists who examined infectious material, such as the contents of smallpox vesicles, had no trouble in perceiving granules, fine globules, and microscopic spheres of different sizes and kinds (including pus globules). Difficulty lay only in determining their significance. Spores and "germs" were readily discovered in smallpox pus and in many other fluids. Henle pointed out, however, that microscopic observations of fungi did not of itself indicate a causal connection.[16] The organisms might be either the result of the disease, or an accidental accompaniment.

By 1840 several instances of *contagium vivum* had been empirically demonstrated. Worm infestations, long familiar, had usually been considered separate diseases rather than causes of disease. The germ theory was not related to parasitism as such but rather to the presence of more minute organisms. The itch mite, identified and recognized as the cause of scabies early in the century, could properly be accounted an animalcule. In 1839 Johann Schoenlein (1793–1864) identified a fungus as the cause of the skin disease favus, and soon the relationship of other specific fungi to other skin diseases was demonstrated.

Fungi could be empirically studied and subjected to experimentation. The existence of bacteria was recognized at that time, but techniques were not available for empirical investigation. There was a vast difference between the general statement: Some diseases are caused by animalcules; and the specific statement: *This* disease is caused by *this* animalcule. The first proposition can readily be accepted as a theory. The latter statement has left the domain of theory and is asserted as a fact. Assertions of fact are much more difficult to accept, especially when they involve so many obscurities.

The modern reader encounters a semantic problem from the

changing meaning of terms and distinctions apparent today but not at all apparent a century and a half ago. Such terms as *vegetable, animal, animalcule, fungus, insect,* and of course, *virus* did not then have the implications current today. The word *animalcule* applied to anything that showed evidence of spontaneous movement, such as spermatozoa, or spirillae, or protozoa, or other organisms seen under the microscope. So too with any structure that manifested growth, multiplication, or "vital" activity. All fell into the category of "little animals." The term *insect* was also used, not in the modern specific taxonomic sense, but rather in the vague connotation of a very small, living, and motile creature.

CONFUSING NOMENCLATURE

In casual remarks, Henle revealed the changes in modes of thinking. When a contagion was first regarded as alive, the human mind, he said, naturally wanted to ascribe to it one of the forms that "the known organic world presents to our senses." In line with this tendency, some individuals "in the earlier childlike period of natural science" guessed at insects. Then he added as if parenthetically, "some simple souls still do so today." However, with gradually increasing knowledge, "it is even more natural to imagine the contagion as having a vegetable body" (ibid., p. 942).

We find this confusing nomenclature remarkably illustrated in the writings of Henry Holland (1788–1873), an influential British physician. He was a sound naturalist, a discursive author, and an outstanding physician with a fashionable and financially rewarding practice. Eventually, his professional eminence was rewarded with knighthood. His numerous and informative essays on various medical topics were published in Great Britain in 1839, with a second edition the next year.[17] We glimpse his breadth of knowledge when we find a footnote in the 1840 edition that mentions Henle's monograph, only just published in Germany (ibid., p. 576). American physicians in the 1840s frequently referred to Holland.

One essay significant for our purposes was entitled in the original edition, "On the Hypothesis of Insect Life as a Cause of Disease?" Holland, however, was definitely not a "simple soul" in the sense that Henle had mentioned. In the third British edition of 1857, reprinted the same year in the United States, the title of this essay was changed to "On the Hypothesis of Animalcule Life as a Cause of Disease?—Cholera." The change from "insect" to "animalcule" indicates a shift in usage, albeit a very slow one.

Well read, Holland represented the armchair theorist, whose insights usually depended on analogy and reasoning. He embraced the animalcular hypotheses, well established by the eighteenth century, that certain disease "derived from minute forms of animal life." He realized, however, that investigation had as yet "furnished nothing beyond stronger presumptions and more numerous analogies" than had been offered in the past (pp. 567–68). He thought it uncertain whether more direct evidence would ever be attained.

To explain the occurrence of explosive epidemics, like the scourge of cholera that had recently swept the world, Holland offered an analogy with "the sudden appearance and multiplication of insect swarms" (p. 584) familiar to naturalists. He also emphasized the role of the atmosphere in the spread of contagion and noted the possibility that "there are germs of life around us, awaiting development" (p. 588).

Holland, an active clinician really belonging to an earlier generation, was well acquainted with recent literature and sympathetic to the animalcular hypothesis. Nevertheless, he maintained a cautious attitude toward evidence. While his professional eminence and his extensive writings helped to promote a climate of opinion favorable to germ theory, he himself did not make any real contribution, either in concrete observations or in critical analysis.

THE INSIGHTS OF JAKOB HENLE

Jakob Henle, on the contrary, was a fine scientist who provided careful analysis and truly clarified some problems of infectious diseases. We recall that the term *miasma* referred to an agent present in the air, while *contagion* referred to an agent that transmitted a disease through contact. The mode of spread had to be kept distinct from the agent itself. Henle distinguished three types of disease, according to the mode of spread. One type was communicated only through the air and never spread by direct contact— it was purely miasmatic. For him, the sole member of this class was the ague. Another type infected exclusively through direct contact; examples were syphilis and scabies. They never spread miasmatically.

The remaining class included those diseases that "appear miasmatically, but apparently are also spread through contagion." These he called "miasmatic-contagious." They included the exanthemata (a group in which scarlatina was deemed a member); "typhoid"; "certain types of cold and catarrh, particularly influenza"; along with dysentery, plague, cholera, and "one form of puerperal fever." To these he added certain localized conditions like ophthalmia neonatorum and hospital gangrene, together with some animal diseases like anthrax.[18] He was referring to the mode and mechanics of spread.

A disease might have a miasmatic origin but could spread by contact. In these conditions, the agent was "a matter which may float in the air as well as be contained in the sick organism . . . and is capable of multiplying within it" (ibid., p. 921). Microscopic examination showed not the agent but only the vehicle with which the agent was associated. The pus within the smallpox vesicle was not the contagion but rather pus *plus* the contagion. The contagion itself was invisible but may have been contained within fluids or have adhered to indifferent objects, known as fomites.

The demonstration of a few infectious agents, and their removal from a hypothetical to an empirical status, did not have much influence on attitudes toward other contagions. The skin diseases caused by fungi were localized, nonfebrile, and had little connection with the febrile diseases that remained so puzzling. And to the average medical mind, a disease of silkworms, if it were known at all, had even less relevance. The role of fungi in a few human diseases did stimulate research but also led to a stronger skepticism. The criteria for proof were becoming more explicit. The presence of particles, granules, and spherules in the fluids of major febrile diseases could lead to assertions and speculations, but eventually an increased empirical and critical attitude would raise new standards of scientific investigation.

The search for specificity continued, but new and critical data were slow in emerging. Meanwhile, physicians tried to arrange and classify the data they had, seeking illumination through analysis.

CLINICAL GROPING TOWARD PRECISE ETIOLOGY

The distinction between the predisposing and the exciting causes became increasingly blurred. Depending on the context, either might serve in the capacity of the other. A different mode of analysis was offered by Charles Williams (1805–69), whose influential text, published in Great Britain in 1843, had an American edition the next year.[19] The book proved extremely popular and by 1853 had achieved its fourth American edition. I have used the first American edition, of 1844.

Williams's analysis tells us much about contemporary thinking and suggests the path that eventually would bring bacteria and comparable agents into the realm of the traditional "exciting causes." He divided all the exciting causes into two classes, the cognizable and the noncognizable. The former identified physical and mental agents of which he believed we have direct awareness. Cold, exertion, and emotion were characteristic examples: we feel a sensation of cold, see muscular exertion, are conscious of "mental emotion." In contrast, noncognizable agents "elude our senses and we infer their existence only from their morbific effects" (ibid., p. 44). For their existence, the evidence was indirect. We might perceive only their manifestations and then postulate the responsible agent.

The ingesta, which he called cognizable agents, illustrate problems that Williams did not appreciate, however apparent they are to us. Ingesta could produce many different kinds of diseases. Irritating substances in food could cause inflammation. Or if "adulterated" (as with lead), the food might act as a poison. Or the ingesta might be deficient in quantity or quality (with a clear reference to our modern deficiency diseases). By calling all these cognizable, Williams implied some directly observed material that represented *the* cause.

Obviously, this is a very loose usage, since what we eat or drink would be merely the vehicle that introduced the actual causal agent into the body. If the ingesta could induce many different diseases, we might assume that separate factors were operative, each of which should be discriminated and identified. Until this degree of specificity was established, the cause could scarcely be regarded as cognizable. Williams, however, did not think in this fashion. A transformation would occur only when the concept of specificity acquired increased importance.

Williams called the second group of agents the noncognizable exciting causes (or poisons) and held them responsible for endemic, epidemic, and infectious diseases. Endemic diseases—like intermittent and remittent fevers—affected persons living in particular areas. The agent was regarded as "an *effluvium, miasm, malaria,* or bad air; an *aerial poison,*" but its nature had not been determined. Despite extensive studies, the poison had not been detected by chemical analysis, and Williams believed that the microscope would eventually discover its nature. Although the nature of the miasma was unknown, some of its "general properties" had been obtained by observing its effects (p. 61). He then enumerated some properties that have been discussed earlier (and which we now know characterize the mosquito).

Other kinds of "malaria" were attracting more and more attention. "There is now abundant evidence that drains, cesspools, and other repositories for effete and putrefying organic matter, evolve exhalations which, when concentrated, may generate low fevers" (p. 61). The "septic" diseases, arising from putrefying organic matter, would become increasingly important for the acceptance of a germ theory.

Epidemic diseases, in contrast to endemic diseases, were not confined to particular localities but might sweep over whole countries in a very short time. The cause was supposedly in the atmosphere, for this constituted "the only thing common to all the places so affected." Some of the epidemic diseases could, Williams thought, be traced to "cognizable qualities" in the air; or to contaminated food, bad water, or other "distinctly cognizable causes." But the varying characteristics of epidemics must be attributed to unknown influences (p. 63).

Williams emphasized that "we are quite in the dark as to the nature of epidemic influences." He did, however, note the "analogical arguments," claiming that "epidemic diseases are caused by animalcule tribes." He referred to the writings of Holland and Henle. He also pointed out the existence of animals and plants acting as parasites in living animals and, in some instances, causing disease. He declared that some epidemic diseases, such as influenza and cholera, "are not inconsistent with the hypothesis that they are caused by the sudden development of animalcules from ova in the blood." However, he went on to say that "there is a total want of direct observation in support of the hypothesis" (p. 64).

We must credit Williams with good critical judgment in holding that the animalcular hypothesis could not be generalized and adopted until better evidence was at hand. However, the older doctrines were showing strains and could no longer be accepted with complacency. Difficulties were becoming apparent.

Disease could be induced by "morbid matter" proceeding from the body of one individual into that of another. Passage could take place through wounds, through (nontraumatic) contact, or through the medium of the air. But regardless of the means, the disease would "propagate its kind." Williams believed that there were only two parallels in nature. One is the case of "septic matter, leaven, or ferment; a little of which introduced into organized matter will promote changes and decompositions." Originally thought to be purely chemical in nature, research had shown that "fermentation is caused by the production and growth of living molecules or vegetables."

Then Williams queried whether "the matter of contagion consist of animal ova or vegetable seeds." In favor of this was the incubation period of many diseases. Furthermore, diseases like scabies or favus were proven examples of parasitism by an animal and a "parasitic vegetable," respectively. However, no such agent was discovered in the lesions of a generalized disease like smallpox. Without such demonstration, "the nature of contagion must remain a matter of speculation" (pp. 66–67). Even if minute animals or "vegetable organisms" had a causal role in some local diseases, generalization of this phenomenon to all infectious diseases was unacceptable without further evidence. Critical judgment demanded caution.

If we go forward a few years we see conceptual progress but not any real empirical advance. Alfred Stillé (1813–1900), a graduate of the University of Pennsylvania in 1836, published a text in 1847 that followed Williams to some extent but offered a greater precision.[20] Like his predecessors, Stillé distinguished predisposing and exciting causes and separated them further into the general and the specific. I will take up only his views on the exciting causes, which he divided into three categories: the general, the special, and the specific.

A general exciting cause gave rise to a disease "without determining either its nature or its seat" (ibid., p. 62), without defining either the location or the character. Thus cold, acting as an excitant, could produce rheumatism or a disturbance of the menstrual cycle. The action would be scarcely separable from a predisposing cause.

Special causes, in contrast, produced definite morbid states but did not furnish unique determinants of the resulting disease. Certain mechanical states, like compressions and obstructions, would be of this type, producing reactions within a limited range. These special causes we would regard as groups of agents that exerted some common type of action but did not themselves determine details.

In this category, Stillé paid much attention to "poisons," of which he enumerated several varieties. He was distinguishing *kinds* of pathogenic activity. Chemical irritants were one kind, "narcotico-acrid" another. This last included certain powerful alkaloids and also "vegetable effluvia," which, by entering the atmosphere, caused hayfever or rose fever.

Especially significant was a group that Stillé designated "septic poisons." These, all generated by putrefaction, could produce "a typhoid or adynamic state," often fatal (p. 93). The poisons might enter the body through food, as "unsound meat or damaged flour"; or through the lungs, if a person were digging in graveyards or sepulchers; or through wounds incurred during anatomical dissection.

This category of "septics" represented a vaguely defined class, whose nature would be elucidated within the next thirty years through bacteriological studies. Stillé placed infectious agents and toxic substances under a single rubric of *septics*, having as a common feature the action of putrefaction. This would form an important part of germ theory. The discrimination of septics would prove to be an important bridge between the earlier animalcular hypothesis and the later science of bacteriology.

Stillé's third category, the specific causes, had unique properties. They "not only engender distinct diseases, but are alone capable of exciting the diseases which follow their application." Their nature and mode of action were unknown, he said, and their very existence was inferred only from the uniformity of their effects and not their actual physical demonstration (pp. 62–63).

Stillé could not resolve the many puzzling features. Some diseases (like syphilis) spread solely by direct contact. Others could spread by direct contact and also through intermediate objects—

fomites. Other diseases spread through "effluvia" in the atmosphere. Of these, intermittent fever never spread by contact, while typhus might do so on occasion. A contagious agent could arise from some effluvia in a spontaneous generation, but other contagions could proceed only from a preexisting agent of the same kind. Some diseases were inoculable, others not. Some diseases were contagious under some circumstances but not under others. They might be capable of being transferred by contact but did not ordinarily act in this way.

These data exemplify a few of the difficulties that attended a causal explanation of disease. At the same time, the "real" nature of a specific agent was not known. Stillé himself emphasized this. John Eberle, in regard to smallpox, referred to the contagious substance "of whose intimate nature and origin we are entirely ignorant." And Elisha Bartlett, speaking of typhoid fever, said that the "essence of the actual, producing, efficient cause . . . are entirely unknown to us."[21]

A specific causal agent could be known by its effects, but its existence was as yet purely hypothetical. Mere armchair reflection on causation could not progress beyond the stage of analogy, which might impress those already sympathetic but carried no real cogency. So too with other indirect evidence, such as epidemiology might furnish. Oliver Wendell Holmes, for example, in his famous paper on the contagiousness of puerperal fever, relied on epidemiology;[22] yet his evidence, although massive, failed to convince the contrary-minded. Reasoning, inference, and indirect evidence would not bring about the conviction that actual empirical demonstration might furnish.

CONTRIBUTIONS FROM OTHER DISCIPLINES

Direct evidence, however, would await the accumulation and digestion of new data. The 1850s and 1860s brought vast expansion in many different areas. One of these dealt with the animalculi as objects of natural history, to be described and classified just as were the larger animal and plant forms. The whole subject of bacterial classification has been well surveyed by William Bulloch.[23]

Microscopy was revealing abundant organisms, especially in putrid and fermenting material. Bacteria and fungi were at first arranged on morphological grounds alone and, because of inadequate culture methods, seemed to change their shape. Primitive culture methods, using only fluid media, might start with one kind of organism but would soon show many different kinds. This led to the concept that fungi and bacteria could readily change their morphology and transform one into another. The specificity of micro-organisms would be recognized only later.

A second major development involved fermentation, wherein Louis Pasteur (1822–95), trained as a chemist, played a leading role.[24] His extensive studies during the 1850s and 1860s did much to establish both the specificity and the functional activity of microorganisms. He showed that specific fermentations would result from specific microorganisms. Another of Pasteur's major contributions in the 1860s was his conclusive refutation of spontaneous generation. He demonstrated that the germs supposedly resulting from spontaneous generation were actually contaminants, living particles that had been floating in the air.

Joseph Lister (1827–1912), trained as a surgeon, saw the implications of Pasteur's work. He appreciated a parallelism between fermentation as a biological process and surgical infection, putrefaction, or gangrene. Furthermore, he believed that the cause of the latter conditions lay with minute particles suspended in the air. These "are the germs of various low forms of life long since revealed by the microscope, and regarded as merely accidental concomitants of putrescence, but now shown by Pasteur to be its essential cause."[25] To control surgical infection, Lister developed his system of "antisepsis" through carbolic acid spray. Originally a practical technique, Lister's work acquired increasing theoretical importance.[26]

At the same time, during the 1850s and 1860s microscopy profoundly affected morbid anatomy and concepts of pathology. Cell theory, blood analysis, investigations of inflammation and the role of the "white corpuscles," experimental work on embolism, the study of "pyemia" as a pathologic phenomenon, and kindred researches, all contributed to a new conceptual framework in which the germ theory would eventually mature. In this framework, new standards were slowly gaining acceptance concerning the criteria for establishing proof and assessing the validity of evidence.

By the early 1870s the whole subject that we now call bacteriology was in turmoil. Each conflicting viewpoint was supported by some sort of experimental evidence. Basic knowledge regarding the natural history of microscopic forms of life had to be acquired slowly, after many false turnings. Moreover, the early technical procedures created many sources of error.

For example, early studies suggested that bacteria were variants of a single type, which could change its form under different circumstances. They had been cultivated in fluid media, such as various vegetable broths, with turnip infusion as a favorite. From a drop of infected material introduced into such an infusion, bacteria would grow rapidly. Within a few days, the population of bacteria would change markedly. Today we recognize the process of contamination. The original inoculum introduced into a broth (which may not have been sterile to begin with) was speedily overgrown by new organisms introduced during manipulation. What we now know as contamination was considered evidence that a single bacterial form could assume different appearances.

For an alternative view, different forms of bacteria would represent different genera and species, subject to appropriate classification. The establishment of specific bacterial types required improved techniques to avoid contamination. Ingenious methods did bring about improvements, but real adequacy would wait until Robert Koch (1843–1910), in the latter 1870s, introduced solid culture media rather than relying solely on broth. It may be noted parenthetically that what we call culture media was at the time described as the "soil" in which the bacteria grew.

AMERICAN INVESTIGATORS GO ASTRAY

During the 1850s and 1860s virtually all original investigations were being carried out in Europe. In the United States, original research was modest indeed, but leading physicians kept up, more or less, with current advances. In the American literature of the early 1870s two especially instructive expositions, by E. P. Hurd and Thomas Satterthwaite, reveal the degree of comprehension prevalent in this country.[27]

Hurd and Satterthwaite, who both wrote shortly before Koch made his epochal discoveries, discussed the knowledge of bacteria at a time when disputes in the European literature were still vigorous. It was only in 1872 that the eminent botanist Ferdinand Cohn (1828–98) propounded his classification of bacteria, and his concepts had by no means generally prevailed. The papers of Hurd and of Satterthwaite vividly reveal the uncertainty surrounding contemporary theory.

Hurd believed in the metamorphosis of microscopic forms. Bacteria seemed to be intermediate between algae and fungi, and he often referred to bacteria as "fungus germs." They would change their form according to the media of growth. Several localized skin diseases could be attributed to fungi as their cause, but these, he maintained, could flourish only in devitalized tissue. "The inoculation of a healthy person with bacteria, or supposed fungus germs, is not necessarily dangerous." Putrefaction (and the germs found therein) might be the result of a disease, and not the cause. (If we do not differentiate one kind from another and do not take account of specificity, we must admit that both of these propositions are clearly true.)

Hurd pointed out that to establish a causal relation it would be needful not merely to recover germs but to produce the disease by injecting them. No generalized (or systemic) infectious disease had yet been traced to bacteria or fungi. He strongly criticized the work of an American physician, J. H. Salisbury, who had attributed the cause of intermittent fever to "vegetable organisms," which he identified as palmellae. The criticisms, which we need not recount here, show a good grasp of critical methodology. Unless we can produce a disease by inoculating the supposed cause, assertion of causal relationship was mere speculation. Scientific work "is inebriated with speculation; the fogs and mists of error blind honest searchers after true knowledge."

Rejecting the germ theory, Hurd embraced the view that "the principle of contagion is a subtle chemical ferment, an organic poison, generated in the body of the diseased individual, derived from other diseased individuals, by infection." In this "chemical view of contagion," a diseased person produced a poison analogous to cobra venom. The poison, when it came in contact with a healthy person, could reproduce the disease. Hurd admitted it would be difficult to isolate such a toxic material from the blood or secretions, yet the difficulties seemed to him less intense than those of conventional germ theory.

At the time, no disease had been definitely linked to bacteria, and there was no compelling distinction that would differentiate bacteria from fungi. To attribute infectious diseases like intermittent fever or typhoid fever to fungi, whatever their form, seemed less credible than attributing them to poisons. Like many investigators, Hurd appreciated the mote in his neighbor's eye but was insensitive to the beam in his own.

The next year, Thomas Satterthwaite, in a detailed paper, also opposed the germ theory, and his arguments reveal the obscurities then prevailing. He affords us glimpses into the contemporary difficulties and the reasons for their genesis. With the background that he furnishes, we can see how Koch's work, carried out within the next few years, solved the problems then at issue.

Satterthwaite objected to the view that "nearly every 'catching' disease is due to a special organism." That such diseases resulted from microscopic bodies was merely an assumption. The alleged causes, the bacteria, might appear in many different forms. He too accepted the current German view of Billroth, that the various forms compose a single entity: just as with fungi, the filaments, hyphae, and spores were all parts of a single organism. Despite their varied appearances, bacteria composed a unity, whose components were more or less equipotential.

Satterthwaite supported his views with several lines of evidence. Thus, one rotten egg might infect another, but he quoted experiments wherein fresh eggs, injected with a fluid that contained bacteria, remained unchanged, "showing, apparently, that bacteria, of themselves, do not necessarily produce decomposition." So too with sepsis. Septic material containing bacteria, when injected into animals, would kill them, and the infection could be transferred from one animal to another. Yet when bacteria alone (that is, not from septic cases) were injected, disease did not necessarily result.

Moreover, bacterial forms were widely present in normal people. "Bacteria which cannot be distinguished . . . from those of disease, have been introduced into the system in numbers without producing any lesions whatever." If bacteria that "cannot be distinguished" were sometimes associated with disease and at other times not, their causal role must remain in doubt. Satterthwaite's conclusions are obviously true, just as long as we do not make any distinction among bacteria.

Satterthwaite discussed at some length the "contagious principles" involved in smallpox, anthrax, relapsing fever (in which a spirillum had only just been observed in the blood in 1872), and typhus. He declared "that we have no reliable evidence that the definite forms described are capable of producing the diseases in question." In smallpox, for example, bacteria might be recovered from the pocks, but any claims of causal relationship were quickly dissipated. The failure with a disease like smallpox strengthened the argument against the causal role of bacteria in general. In retrospect, we see that progress would depend on establishing the specificity of bacteria and the differences in properties.

CANONS OF PROOF: ROBERT KOCH

Before presenting the evidence that would soon be forthcoming, I would comment on the notion of specificity. As we have seen, the subject had long been a matter of interest, but attention had focused on the specificity of diseases as clinical entities. In the eighteenth century, physicians sought the clinical (and even anatomical) features that would sharply mark one disease from another. Considerable progress had been made since the early nosologists first devoted themselves to this task. In the nineteenth century, the emphasis gradually shifted. The problems took a new form. Instead of asking, What makes diseases clinically specific?, physicians asked, rather, To what extent are the *causes* of disease specific? Specificity remained the chief problem but in a different locus of investigation.

A new dimension was intruding itself in regard to causation. Since antiquity, physicians had tried to explain phenomena through their causes, but the problems had not been really troublesome when the explanations rested on hypothetical entities like Boerhaave's "acrimomy" or "spissitude."[28] These, as alleged causes, were not matters of empirical observation. By the mid-nineteenth century, however, physicians could point to material objects, like fungi and bacteria, and assert that these caused disease. Bacteria were empirically observable, not conceptual or hypothetical.

The problem changed. Did these observable entities in fact

cause the disease in question? Physicians had to wrestle with the questions, What constitutes a fact? How do you establish it? To what inferences does it give rise? Is an asserted causal connection really a fact? These, of course, were not new problems, but by the third quarter of the nineteenth century they had acquired a special urgency. And physicians were not well equipped to handle them.

Robert Koch did much to strengthen the ties between medicine and the philosophy of science, a topic to which I will return in the next chapter. Koch brought to the problems of medicine a fabulous degree of technical expertise and at the same time a clear perception of logical pitfalls and ways to avoid them. After perceiving the essence of a problem, he devised technical means to reach a solution. At the same time, he clarified the philosophic and logical implications. Biographical details and an overview of his life work are well presented in histories of bacteriology already referred to.[29]

His first great scientific triumph, in 1876 (published in 1877), related to anthrax, a disease in which previous studies had not achieved conclusive results. Earlier workers had transmitted the disease by inoculations of blood and had shown, moreover, that blood contained abundant bacteria. But other students of the subject failed to transmit the disease with blood that contained bacteria, while still others claimed to have succeeded with bacteria-free blood.

Koch's own contributions were in large part technical and methodological, but they also related to his broad conceptions of biological problems. With great virtuosity and under difficult circumstances, he devised new methods as the need arose. Starting with the blood of animals with anthrax, he was able to isolate the bacteria, grow them in a pure culture, and study their life cycle under the microscope. He demonstrated the formation of spores and showed that these could change back into the vegetative form and cause the disease. Repeated passages through animals always ended up with the identical bacteria. However, different test animals (mice, guinea pigs, and rabbits) would show differences in the distribution of the organisms, and bacteria might be demonstrable in some tissues but not in the blood.

Koch declared that he had, for the first time, "established the etiology of anthrax." Typhoid fever and cholera, which he declared similar to anthrax in their mode of dissemination, might also be due to bacteria. But even if such organisms were found, "we would still be hampered by the fact that these diseases do not occur in animals." In this early work, we can see steps that led to his famous postulates. In the next chapter, I will consider in detail the concepts involved.

Koch's second major contribution dealt with sepsis, which, as we have seen, posed certain problems in theories of causation. Putrid, decomposing, or septic material, when injected into animals, would prove fatal. At first this had been regarded as a toxic manifestation, the effect of a poison. Earlier writers, as we have seen, regarded sepsis as if it were a unit. When later studies showed that septic material contained bacteria varying widely in morphology, the question arose concerning their causative role. Scientists who were denying the specificity of bacterial types might continue to regard sepsis as a unitary process.

Ferdinand Cohn and others maintained that essential differences existed between bacterial types and implied the existence of functional as well as morphological variation. Logic demanded that such bacterial types, if truly distinct, should induce demonstrably different diseases. In the 1870s, prior to the work of Koch, this had never been demonstrated. Koch investigated blood and broth cultures that had putrefied, as well as material from gangrene, abscesses, pyemia, septicemia, and erysipelas. For his experiments he used chiefly mice and rabbits. The septic material of different origins would kill experimental animals, and Koch could recover different kinds of bacteria. After serial passages, the bacteria recovered from experimental animals remained true to type—metamorphosis did not occur.

In his researches, Koch went far beyond mere morphological specificity. He also emphasized the need to study "physiological effects such as character of spread in tissues, types of cell attacked, and toxic effects," that is, the way the particular bacterial form behaved, in a biological sense (ibid., p. 82). Specificity depended on far more than shape and size.

Through his inoculation experiments, Koch succeeded in showing that different sources of septic material, which superficially might seem similar, yielded specific kinds of bacteria. Moreover, he could maintain these in a pure culture in animals through successive passages, always producing the same disease and, after many transfers, end with the same type as that with which he started.

The host animal might serve as a means of achieving a pure culture of bacteria and of separating out mixtures of organisms. As an example, he pointed to putrefying blood. This, on direct microscopic observation, contained a great variety of bacteria, but Koch declared that only two types could survive and grow in the laboratory mouse. One was a small bacillary form, causing "septicemia"; and the other, a coccus that caused "gangrene." These two could, however, be separated by inoculation into mice in whom the bacilli disappeared while the cocci multiplied.

This work of Koch of 1878 I consider, in a sense, his most important contribution, although not his most dramatic. He showed that "sepsis," or "gangrene," or putrefying matter comprehended many separable conditions, each with an identifiable causative agent. Particular agents, through appropriate technical means, could be separated and maintained in pure culture, as pathogenic organisms. He established the specificity of bacterial types and included their functional and biological behavior among their characteristics to be studied, in addition to their morphological features. He contributed to the problem of host specificity, which in experimental work would become increasingly important as time went on. And from the standpoint of scientific method, this paper furnished the major support for his so-called postulates. He laid the perfect groundwork for the study of tuberculosis.

Koch's study of anthrax showed for the first time that a human disease had as its cause a specific bacterium. But anthrax was not a very important disease, and most practitioners regarded it with little concern. Similarly, the investigation of sepsis had but slight impact on the medical profession as a whole. Far different, however, was the reaction to Koch's discovery of the tubercle bacillus and his flawless proof that this was indeed the "cause" of the disease. The discovery, announced in 1882, electrified the medical world.

Elsewhere I have discussed at some length the problems of tuberculosis and the part that Koch played.[30] Suffice here to mention only a few of the salient features. Physicians had long disputed whether tuberculosis was an infectious disease. By 1868 the French investigator Jean Antoine Villemin (1827–92) succeeded in showing experimentally that he could transmit the disease from humans to animals by inoculation. The identity of the natural and the experimental diseases was shown by anatomical studies. But even when the disease was shown to be contagious, the nature of the agent—the "contagion"—could not be demonstrated.

Through his innovations in straining technique, Koch was able to demonstrate the bacillus, histologically, in every case of the disease. Furthermore, through further technical innovations, he was able to culture the bacterium free of all contaminants. Then, by injecting a pure culture into test animals, he elicited the clinical and anatomical features of tuberculosis—he had "reproduced the disease." Apart from offering new technical procedures, Koch's work of 1882 provided rigorous criteria of proof that would apply to any alleged cause for an infectious disease.[31]

AMERICAN DISCIPLES OF KOCH

Koch's announcement had a profound effect the world over, yet in the United States the subject of bacteriology was not well appreciated. Koch's achievements have to be placed in context. In February and March 1883, less than a year after Koch's announcement regarding tuberculosis, a young Chicago physician, William Belfield, who had been studying in Germany, gave a series of four lectures in New York. These, originally published in the *Medical Record*, were reprinted as a book in 1884.[32] Belfield was trying not so much to publicize Koch's latest discovery as to acquaint the "busy practitioner" with "facts which he has not time to seek, amid the mass of current literature" (ibid., p. 115). As part of this program, Belfield offered a broad survey of prevailing concepts regarding bacteria, their morphology, classification, and properties.

The lectures, however, are not a mere account of scientific advances. Much of the text is given over to censorious remarks concerning research in America and the level of bacterial knowledge. He condemned, with much sarcasm, physicians who knew very little about bacteria but nevertheless loudly expressed their opinions, founded on ignorance. The book has unexpected value, for it depicts by indirection the general state of ignorance in the medical community, the slow diffusion of new scientific knowledge, and the inability to evaluate evidence.

Belfield did not offer a systematic exposition of erroneous views but scattered his remarks among his own expositions. Some of his comments reflect the American milieu in the early 1880s. Belfield himself, highly elitist, was strongly critical of those who offered strong opinions without adequate training. In this country, he said, there were "at present perhaps a score of men who have given abundant evidence of competence in bacterial investigation," and it is to these men, "not to dermatologists, surgeons, or pathologists, we must look for facts upon this subject" (p. 28). He devoted much time to Koch's methods and stressed the difference between facts and opinion, between demonstration and assertion.

Belfield also emphasized the difference between good and bad research. Koch's demonstration regarding anthrax was "so clear and unequivocal as to convince skepticism and silence casuistry. It is, therefore, the rock . . . on which the bacteriologists seek refuge from the waves of ridicule" (p. 64). Some of the book is devoted to explaining the difference between good and bad science. Because much research, in this country and in Europe, had proven so inadequate, popular scorn had attacked the view that bacteria caused disease. "There is a gentleman in this State who recently reminded us that bacteria, so-called, are in his opinion fibrin threads . . . and there is said to be a man in Virginia who insists that the earth is flat" (pp. 79–80).

The lectures, with their incidental comments, let us glimpse the prevailing status of the principles of bacteriology. As a clinical example, Belfield mentioned a surgeon performing a laparotomy who used carbolic spray: hands, ligatures, and instruments were "thoroughly carbolized." However, the skin was not even washed, and coils of intestine came in contact with pubic hair. The patient died of peritonitis (pp. 55–56). Belfield explained the principles that would prevent infection, including not only cleanliness but meticulous surgical technique, with ligation of vessels and the elimination of necrotic tissue in which bacteria might grow.

The book wandered rather discursively. It explained the new data of bacteriology, especially the work of Koch, with special emphasis on his methods of proof. Then it tried to induce an awareness of bacteriological principles. It also tried to raise the level of research and study and expressed great hopes for the future. "But these results can be secured only by earnest, skilful, continuous experimental investigation, which is practically impossible without pecuniary support" (p. 114). And he pointed to the governmental support offered in France and Germany.

Quite different is H. Gradle's book, an orderly presentation of bacteriology as then known.[33] It was a true textbook on the subject, along the lines of a French text that George Sternberg translated in 1880.[34] This latter volume of 189 pages gave a historical account of experimental work, described what was known of bacteria and their properties, and noted their possible role in various diseases, including anthrax, smallpox, measles, diphtheria, and typhoid fever. We know now that, except for anthrax, all the claims were erroneous. For anthrax, the author stated cautiously that Koch's work (of 1876) added "an additional element of probability in favor of parasitic theory" (ibid., p. 161). Gradle's book, quite comparable, was written several years later and hence could incorporate newer findings. Koch's work received good coverage and needs no further discussion here. I will, however, mention the presentation of two other diseases, typhoid fever and diphtheria.

PROGRESS IN BACTERIOLOGY

Gradle noted that many observers had described bacteria in typhoid fever. He paid special attention to the work of Carl Eberth who, in 1880, described a special bacillus observed in stained sections of tissues. (Actually, the organism had been noted earlier, by Koch, who had photomicrographs of his findings.) This organism, not cultured until 1884, is now accepted as the infectious agent, and was named after Carl Eberth, but when Gradle wrote there was no proof. He declared, "the causal relation of the parasite to the disease can of course not be affirmed until proven by inoculation experiments."[35]

Regarding diphtheria, Gradle was even more critical. Many different bacteria had been noted and cultured, but Gradle emphasized the lack of proof. He mentioned Arnold Klebs, who even then had a dubious reputation. Gradle commented that Klebs "had by this time discovered the germs of almost every disease" (ibid., p. 190), including typhoid fever. For diphtheria, he had already discovered a "micrococcus diphthericus." Ironically, in 1883 Klebs did describe the bacillus that became accepted as the cause, but the proof was established in 1884 by Friedrich Loeffler, who conducted fine cultural and inoculation experiments. The designation Klebs-Loeffler bacillus gives credit to both men, and compensates Klebs for all the times he was so abysmally wrong.

When Gradle published his book, the "golden age of bacteriology" was still developing, and his text gives us a good glimpse of what was going on. Progress was indeed rapid, as shown in a review article that James T. Whittaker published in 1886.[36] He called it merely, "Some Points in Bacteriology," but today it might include the words "Recent Advances." These were so profound, he said, that the medical curriculum should make obligatory at least a three-months' course in bacteriology.

The relation of specific bacteria to specific diseases was established, and now the characteristics and relationships of bacteria— what we might call their life history—were being studied. Variations in morphology, including colony forms; attenuation of pathogenic properties; chemical reactions; cultural requirements and reaction to various culture media (or soils, in the contemporary usage); modes of differentiating bacteria that might seem similar; cellular reactions induced in the host; a rudimentary approach to immunity—these are a few of the topics on which Whittaker commented. When elaborated, they would characterize bacteriology as an independent discipline.

He was, he declared, merely indicating the research that "the most advanced observers" had been carrying out in the past year or so. He held out a rosy prospect for the future, looking forward to the time when "practitioners of medicine [will] no longer be compelled to rely on raw empiricism." Instead, by investigating specific causes, they might be able to find specific remedies.

Some practitioners, however, regarded all this as more or less an ivory tower, of no practical value. At the annual meeting of the American Medical Association, the chairman of the Medical Section had the task of describing the "progress during the past year in materia medica and the practice of medicine." In 1885 the chairman of the section was Henry D. Didama, a colorful figure prominent in medical politics. He offered a point of view rather different from Whittaker's.[37]

Accepting, perhaps a little grudgingly, the asserted causal relations between bacteria and diseases, Didama discussed at some length the recent work on cholera. Koch had recently (1884) identified the "comma bacillus" as the causative agent. With purple rhetoric, Didama praised the zeal and courage of investigators and the sacrifices they made. Then in the same vein he queried, "Does not truth compel the sad confession that bacteriology, with all its brilliant discoveries, has furnished little help to what is of the greatest practical importance to physicians and patients, the art of healing?" The discoveries had not checked the progress of the diseases, nor modified treatment. Improved therapy in cholera had been successfully used "more than a decade of years before it was known whether the cause of the disease was shaped like a comma or an interrogation point."

Nevertheless, Didama did maintain the value of science. "Let the spirit of inquiry suffer no discouragement." In some way, research might help prevent and cure disease. But, he asked, might he not suggest to investigators "that the shape of the microbes, or even their behavior in cultivation fluids, is no longer of supreme importance?"

Ironically, within a few years events showed that Didama had chosen unfortunate subjects for his rhetoric. In talking about shapes of bacteria, he specifically mentioned the "micrococcus of diphtheria," a clear reference to Klebs's earlier and misguided claims of causation. But virtually while Didama was speaking, Loeffler, working with a bacillus that Klebs had newly described in diphtheria, developed staining techniques (as well as culture methods) that offered everything Didama could possibly have wanted. The morphology of bacteria (the shape, which to Didama had little importance) proved highly significant in diagnosis and treatment and established the concrete practical value of bacteriology.

Loeffler's staining techniques and his method of rapid cultivation made identification of the diphtheria bacillus relatively easy for the trained worker. This identification, however, depended on special techniques beyond the scope of the practicing physician. As early as 1886, Boston City Hospital set aside a special room for the laboratory diagnosis of diphtheria.[38]

Rapid diagnosis happened to mesh with advances in the realm of immunology that were emerging in the 1880s. Different lines of research blended perfectly. In diphtheria, lesions were found to result from a toxin that the bacteria produced. In the budding field of immunology, investigators sought ways to neutralize the toxin and thus provide a means of combatting the disease. Many workers attacked the problem, but major credit belongs to Emil von Behring and S. Kitasato, who succeeded in immunizing animals against the toxin. The blood of these animals contained antitoxin, which could protect nonimmune animals against injections of toxin.

This work, published in 1890, led to the successful treatment of the human disease with antitoxin. In 1891 the first human patient with diphtheria received antitoxin, and by the next year commercial production became feasible.[39] Germ theory, interacting with concepts of specificity and causation, had developed methods whose practical value was incalculable and that would transform medicine in both its practical and theoretical aspects.

GERM THEORY AND ITS EFFECTS ON CLINICAL PRACTICE

I close this chapter with a few details regarding practice, and in the next chapter I deal with the broader conceptual transformations and interrelationships. In the 1890s, the significance of laboratory study was diffusing slowly but surely and at the same time inducing massive changes in practice. In 1893 a physician, in discussing diphtheria, noted the difficulties in diagnosing the disease on purely clinical grounds and the harm that could come from a wrong diagnosis. However, he commented, "not long ago science came to our aid," and the Klebs-Loeffler bacillus was recognized as the characteristic and pathognomonic finding.

Yet most clinicians could not make the necessary examination, for "only a few of our young members have had the advantage of such training in special laboratory courses."[40]

In New York, he pointed out, the Board of Health provided, free of charge, the appropriate laboratory tests. In three months, 431 cultures had been examined, of which 301 were positive. The author pleaded for widespread extension of such diagnostic facilities. The paper made no mention of antitoxin and its potential role.

Within the next two years, the situation had changed substantially. An editorial in JAMA declared, "So firmly is the bacteriological diagnosis test relied upon, that communities and boards of health all over the world are establishing expensive laboratories mainly for the purpose of making these culture tests for K-L bacillus."[41]

Furthermore—and perhaps nothing could be more "practical" for some physicians—"in thus coming to the aid of the physician, the authorities formally relieve him of the risk and responsibility of making the positive diagnosis of diphtheria." The editorial cited a lawsuit for $50,000 brought against a physician for faulty diagnosis. A report from a public health laboratory, said the editorial, "would have a very soothing influence upon the mind of the doctor defendant."

8

Changing Aspects of Scientific Medicine, 1800–1850

PRESENT-DAY AMERICAN CULTURE TAKES GREAT PRIDE in its scientific medicine, but when historians want to know just what this really means, they encounter much confusion. Two exceedingly complex terms, *science* and *medicine*, have been conjoined and, as a result, have expanded their individual complexities.

Science has several components. One of them is theory, which I regard as a systematic aggregate of concepts that serve an explanatory function. In medicine the explanatory concepts have always reflected the science of the day. Thus, the "faculties" of Galen or the "mercury" of Paracelsus arose from contemporary science, just as do the viruses and genes of today. This explanatory (or conceptual) aspect, drawn from contemporary science, plays its role in scientific medicine.

Science also claims a validity for its various pronouncements, but how do we know that the doctrines are really well founded? Explanatory theories depend on evidence, and this evidence must be evaluated. Today we speak confidently of experimental design, controls, single and double blind, bias, and statistical analysis—ways of making sure that the assertions are reliable. Earlier historical eras also had criteria for justifying assertions—rather different, however, from those current today. All these various modes, present and past, compose the methodology of science, which may be summed up as critical attitude.

Besides the conceptual and methodological aspects of science, there is a third, which I call the technological component. It refers to the use of tools to provide greater discrimination. A simple example is a magnifying glass; an instance a little more complex would be a stethoscope; and one still more so, an x-ray machine. The history of technology is a fascinating discipline in its own right. For medicine, the best and most compendious account of technical improvements is Stanley Reiser's book.[1]

In medicine we have always had a further complexity—the division into theory and practice (sometimes called science and art). The one has primarily to do with understanding, the other with therapy. Often the two reinforce each other, so that the better the understanding of nature, the more effective the therapy. Sometimes, however, the two components go each its separate way, with little interaction.

When we speak of scientific medicine, we must keep in mind just what we are talking about. Practitioners who call on sophisticated technology in practice may be quite ignorant of theory. Or they may know a great deal of theory but be quite uncritical of the way they apply it. Or, perhaps, research physicians who make conceptual advances may be dismally incompetent if they try to treat patients. These ambiguities complicate the term *scientific medicine*. Its different facets, while perhaps all ultimately interrelated, developed at different rates and under different influences.

In this confused area, Benjamin Rush had one view of what scientific medicine meant, William Osler quite another. To analyze the transition and to provide a suitable framework for discussion, I will go back to the concept of empiricism and the changes in meaning that it underwent.

DIFFERENT MEANINGS OF EMPIRICISM

In most of the eighteenth century, *empiricism* was a pejorative term, implying an ignorance of medical theory (i.e., of science). However, by the early nineteenth century two distinct and opposite influences were affecting this attitude.

On the one hand, the growing spirit of analysis and experimentation gave a heightened value to experience and was making the term *empiricism* not only respectable but worthy of high praise. It replaced rationalism as the proper methodological approach.

However, other influences tended to preserve the older usage. The increasingly popular medical sects, such as homeopathy and Thomsonianism, had rejected the conceptual basis of regular medicine and, by their ignorance of (orthodox) medical theories, were empirics by definition. These sects kept alive the pejorative sense of *empiricism.*

Additional confusion arose from the sad state of medical education, wherein some schools turned out extremely ignorant practitioners, who had the M.D. degree but whose knowledge of medical science was negligible. These men were empirics in the eighteenth century sense, indicating an ignorance of science.

The two senses of *empiricism,* involving both good and bad, played a considerable part in the history of American medicine. By mid-nineteenth century, leading physicians were emphasizing experience in its good sense, and by the end of the century a new canon of scientific method had taken root. Nevertheless, the term *empiricism* still remained a "bad word" when applied to those practitioners who did not heed the "new" science.

The changing criteria of what constituted science can readily be traced back to Francis Bacon in the seventeenth century. He made no discoveries and did not advance the substantive aspects of science. He did, however, formulate a methodology that developed into the modern scientific method.[2] In the early nineteenth century, advances in medical science were commonly associated with so-called positivism. This movement, which indirectly influenced American medicine, is usually connected with August Comte (1798–1857). Actually, it represents the whole growth of empirical philosophy, whose modern development from Francis Bacon (1561–1626) through John Locke (1632–1704) and Dugald Stewart (1753–1828) strongly affected leading American physicians.[3]

The difference between medical empiricism and medical rationalism is only a matter of degree and emphasis, for neither doctrine can exist without the other.[4] A working synthesis was achieved by William Cullen, whose views dominated American medicine in the eighteenth century. However, Benjamin Rush, his most prominent disciple in America, introduced severe distortions.

In medicine, the explosive growth of empirical method (in its good sense) during the nineteenth century occurred chiefly in

France. For almost half a century, French medicine truly dominated the entire medical world. For this period, Erwin Ackerknecht's study is the only overall survey, but his evaluations must be regarded cautiously.[5] In presenting the contrapuntal relationships of the old and the new, I do not attempt any systematic coverage. Instead, I focus on the men who, in my opinion, best illustrate certain problems and the stages of gradual resolution.

SAMUEL JACKSON AND THE NEW EMPIRICAL PHILOSOPHY

Samuel Jackson (1787–1872) has been generally neglected by medical historians. He received his medical degree from the University of Pennsylvania in 1808 and was entirely American trained.[6] He joined the medical faculty as a lecturer in the institutes of medicine and later succeeded to the chair in that subject.

A prolific author, Jackson wrote an important book in 1832 whose preface contained a splendid digest of current medical philosophy.[7] The book expounded not the practice of medicine but its "principles" as contained in the institutes of medicine. When he wrote, this subject had come to represent chiefly physiology rather than the whole field of medical science, as had been the case in the eighteenth century. Jackson, I may say parenthetically, was a vitalist.

Although not at all an investigator, Jackson was extremely well read. For the preparation of his book, he acknowledged indebtedness to Haller, Bichat, Broussais, Gendrin, and Andral, among others (ibid., p. xx). I would emphasize that Louis does not appear in this list; however, when discussing the relatively new "organic medicine," Jackson included Louis among his sources.

Jackson also published many Introductory Lectures, given over the years for his course in the institutes of medicine. These lectures afforded him an opportunity to express a personal philosophy, not necessarily related directly to the subject matter of the course but still indicative of various problems important at the time. For the present discussion, the lecture of 1833 is especially relevant.[8]

In his textbook, Jackson wanted to indicate to his students "the line of march now taken up by the science of medicine." In so doing he noted the low status of medical practice. It rested on experience, and this, he emphasized, was a questionable guide. Because individuals and circumstances might vary so greatly, experience in medicine could never yield the assurance that experience yielded in other sciences, which, according to Dugald Stewart, one could "predict with almost infallible certainty."[9] Medicine, Jackson went on, was not an art "preceptive" in character, that is, to be acquired merely by learning rules and principles. (This was the essence of empiricism.) Rather, medicine was a demonstrative science, subject to the rules of causality.

Uncertainty, which had become a reproach in medicine, had originally applied to all science "before the introduction of positive philosophy." If this philosophy were applied to medicine, there could result "a degree of certainty" difficult to grasp at that moment.

Francis Bacon, he said, had discovered "the true method of philosophizing, by means of experiment and induction," and by depending on nature rather than authority. Nevertheless, in medicine, authority had long prevailed and had "shed abroad its disastrous influence. It has retarded and must continue to shackle the progress of our science." All this would change "when authority is discarded and analysis, or positive philosophy, preside over science" (ibid., p. xiii).

This view, of course, had long been approved. In the seventeenth century, the Royal Society of London had explicitly adopted the same concept in its motto, *Nullius in Verbis*. Physicians, even those generally regarded as rationalists, had also accepted it on a verbal level. By the nineteenth century, physicians who had hitherto honored Bacon in the breach rather than in the observance were no longer content with mere lip service. They began actually to apply Bacon's doctrines.

Comte struck an agreeable chord when he arranged the sciences according to their degree of certainty, which in turn was related to subject matter. Most precise were mathematics. Then came astronomy, then physics, then chemistry, then the sciences of living matter, which for medicine meant physiology. Despite differing degrees of certainty, the positive method was applicable in all. Medicine should be investigated in the same manner as chemistry and physics, "by the experimental, analytic, and inductive method applied to all the subjects of its inquiry and research" (p. xiv).

Through the inductive method, "general conclusions" could be ascertained and, if confirmed "by repeated experience and diversified observation, they may be adopted as principles capable of a safe and sound application." Three different types of principles (or "methods") had been successively adopted. First was symptomatic medicine, in which diseases were regarded as groups of symptoms, and these alone demanded therapy. (This usage persists today in the expression symptomatic treatment.) Second was organic medicine. In this mode, the symptoms were "traced up to their causes," namely, the organs giving rise to the symptoms. And third was physiological medicine. Here physicians recognized that the essential character of disease resided in "the physiological or vital action of the tissues" (pp. xiv, xv).

Organic medicine, Jackson pointed out, with its dependence on pathology (i.e., morbid anatomy), had developed chiefly in Paris, with its many large hospitals. Jackson mentioned the great contributors, including Bayle, Laennec, Andral, Gendrin, and Louis among the French physicians, and Bright and Forbes among the British. He lamented the virtual absence of American names. This he attributed to "the paucity of hospitals, and the miserable arrangements, as regards the great interests of science, under which they are placed. Until the facilities of investigation are freely granted to the medical profession in these institutions, organic medicine cannot flourish in this country" (p. xvii).

Through the autopsy, organic medicine could demonstrate to the senses the structural alterations occurring in disease. But these alterations were themselves effects, produced by an antecedent cause that was physiological in nature. To achieve certainty in medicine, the physician must determine the characteristic features of these physiological phenomena. This reduced itself to "the nature of the vital actions and phenomena—the reaction of the organism to impressions," and the laws that they follow.

This represented true physiological medicine. Jackson pointed out that earlier systems of medicine had also been truly physiological, but the physiological ideas of earlier times had been defective— "mere collections of hypotheses." The "facts" on which physicians relied had been "imperfect" and often only "hypothetical." In the present state of medical knowledge, the safest course was to generalize the facts but "with a cautious spirit, under the guidance of analysis and induction" (pp. xviii–xix).

THE RELATION OF "FACTS" AND "PRINCIPLES"

Jackson had learned his lesson well. Without making any original contribution of his own, he was presenting to the American public some ideas that had developed, largely in France, since the turn of the century. The ideas were not the product of any one investigator but instead permeated the intellectual environment as a "spirit of the times." Before we examine the further development, we must note Jackson's views on "fact."

Difficulties in science, he said, arise from the dependence on alleged facts that turn out to be wrong—what he called "false facts." Facts by themselves—whether true or false—were of no use. They had value only "as they enable us to determine principles, and to institute theories; and if we err in theories, it is, either that the facts are imperfectly known,—or, what is furnished us as fact, are false."[10]

Yet even when reliable facts were abundantly present, the implications did not automatically emerge. Genius was required to make generalizations and to establish "a sound theory of universal applicability." Such genius "immediately perceives the similarities and resemblances of things; embraces, analyzes, and distinguishes the slightest particularities of objects . . . and deduces from the study of their general relations, their reciprocal connection and mutual dependence, the causes or laws regulating their production" (ibid.). The phrase "aha reaction" was not as yet current at that time, but Jackson was obviously referring to the same sort of sudden insight implied by that modern phrase.

Facts, he said, are not science but only the material of science. The latter had no existence "until principles are evolved, or theory is perfected." The facts were known through the medium of the senses, but they must be arranged through the reflecting powers of the mind. The connection (i.e., the causality) between facts must be discovered (ibid., p. 16). Generalization represented an active process. Furthermore, contrary to the view of Bacon, a suitable arrangement of facts did not place all wits on a level.

The great question remained, what constitutes a fact and how is it determined? Jackson's answer: a fact "is a simple indivisible phenomenon, presented by a natural phenomenon, ascertained by the senses by careful observation, tested by the experience of thousands, the same in all ages, and verified by reiterated experiments." Unfortunately, he said, only a few of the facts in medicine were of this character. Too often a single observation, in a single case, was hastily announced to be a fact and from it a "practical precept" (i.e., a therapeutic indication) was "falsely deduced." Such an "unphilosophical" procedure had overwhelmed medicine with "false facts" (p. 19).

Jackson also indicated, although somewhat obscurely, what he meant by "principles." Natural phenomena, he said, might be classified according to their resemblances and differences. If groupings "in their essential circumstances, are exactly the same [they] have the same cause, and constitute one fact." This primary fact represented a generalization, that is, the "concentration" of many facts into one. Such a "general fact is a principle from which, all the series of phenomena below it, arise immediately or secondarily" (p. 19). In this rather confusing formulation, I glimpse a vague residue of Platonism and the doctrine of universals, all set in a realist philosophy.[11]

Jackson was admittedly an eclectic. Certainly, when we examine his views on the nature of medical science, we can clearly perceive elements already expressed by Francis Bacon, John Locke, Herman Boerhaave, and William Cullen, as well as the French positivists. Jackson added nothing new, but he did formulate and systematize the thinking of the era. No American physician had previously presented these views to his fellow physicians in a manner equally explicit and straightforward.

Although Jackson emphasized the importance of "true" facts, he did not offer any practical method for testing their validity. He gave no concrete suggestions for improving the reliability of medical data. His discussion on a verbal level did not help the students to whom the lecture was directed. This defect resulted directly from his lack of experience in investigative work. He was really an eighteenth-century thinker, although well tinctured by later influences. Actually, he provided little concrete advance over William Cullen, who also greatly admired Francis Bacon. In essence, Jackson brought Cullen's views up to date.

With the example of Samuel Jackson before us, we can better appreciate the views of Pierre Louis, with their advances and their retrogressions, and their widespread influence in the United States.

PIERRE LOUIS AND HIS NUMERICAL METHOD

It was William Osler's essay on Louis that alerted modern historians of American medicine to the importance of this seminal physician.[12] Elsewhere in this book I have dealt with certain aspects of his thinking, especially in relation to typhoid fever. Here I want to discuss his contributions to scientific medicine.

By coincidence, Louis was an exact contemporary of Jackson. Louis, however, working in a markedly different environment, was actually participating in movements and trends that Jackson could only read about. Louis's own great contribution concerned the need for precision and accuracy in the collection of facts. He advanced the methodology of science rather than its theory or technology. Although Jackson and Louis both recognized the need for "true" facts, only Louis provided a technique for assuring their validity.

In developing his methodology, he emphasized observation, precision, accuracy, and quantitation, all codified in the popular term *numerical method*. With minute care, he studied patients on the wards, taking detailed notes on their history, physical examination, treatment, and clinical course. If the patient died, Louis performed an autopsy with a similar degree of precision. Quite aware that his methods departed from current modes of clinical study, he described his procedures in some detail. For the contemporary American medical public, he provided some methodological details in his book on phthisis. A memoir published in French, and translated into English in 1838, went into much greater detail. James Jackson, who wrote the preface to Louis's book on bloodletting, also described the method at some length.[13]

Medicine, said Louis, was a science of observation, and each patient posed a separate problem, for whose solution "we must collect the greatest number of data that we possibly can." In studying the patient, the proper procedure was "to make inquiries relative to *all* the functions during life, to describe *all* the organs after death, and ... [then] analyze them with care, and deduce what consequences we can." The imperfections of the current medical science resulted from analyses that were incomplete or that depended on facts entrusted to memory rather than to careful records.[14] Louis wanted to change all that.

When collecting facts about a patient, Louis noted the differing degrees of reliability. Most objective, he thought, was direct personal observation. Less reliable were the data elicited through questioning. When interrogating a patient, he asked their age; occupation; diet; changes in state of health, especially of nutrition; past illnesses, including their origin, duration, and the order in which symptoms developed; and a detailed account of bodily functions. All this resembles the routine impressed on present-day medical students, when first learning to take a clinical history. Data, said Louis, were reliable only when derived from patients "endowed with a certain share of understanding, and more especially of memory."[15] Raw data had to be critically evaluated before they could be accepted.

Louis wanted "all" the facts, since a physician cannot draw correct conclusions unless he takes into account "all the data which can, or ought to, enter into the solution of the problem."[16] Similarly, when performing an autopsy (which required at least two hours), he described as accurately as possible "the situation, form, colour, consistence, and thickness of organs . . . in a word, all the changes they presented."[17] He held the naive belief that he could actually encompass "all" the data.

The nonoccurrence of a lesion or symptom might prove just as significant as its presence. However, only a specific notation, made at the time of examination, would constitute reliable evidence of presence or absence. Vague recollection was in no sense the equivalent of explicit documentation made at the time of examination.

The facts, after they had been gathered, must be analyzed and arranged according to their resemblances. To this end Louis, with great labor, constructed tables that would display various features and relationships, such as incidence, similarities and differences, course, duration, and associated conditions. Such listings of presence or absence would, he thought, display the essential features of a disease. How happy he would have been with our modern computers!

The frequency with which clinical or anatomical findings occurred must be known precisely to permit exact percentages. This involved counting. "Between him who counts, in order to analyze rigorously, and him who has not counted and who uses the expressions more or less, rare or frequent, there is all the difference that there is between day and night, truth and error."[18] Louis condemned vague assertions that a particular treatment would "often" cure the patient. What did "often" mean? Proper observation required precise enumeration of reliable data, which must be critically examined for validity.

We may fairly ask, What did Louis's method, elaborated in the 1820s, really accomplish? With his accumulated masses of data, he helped circumscribe diseases such as typhoid fever or phthisis, and by detailing the incidence of various factors, he allowed a more precise description. He established standards of accuracy, and was effective as a teacher.

But Louis himself did not make any important discoveries. Tabulation of data, painstakingly collected, did not substitute for new insight. To use Samuel Jackson's phrase, Louis had far less "genius" than did, say, Pierre Brettonneau, who was also a good observer. Yet Brettonneau made his discoveries without Louis's almost neurotic compulsion to accumulate data. However, if anyone had questioned his conclusions and asked that devastating question, But how do you know? Louis could have offered "facts" to justify his claims.

TESTING THE EFFICACY OF BLOODLETTING

Louis's method found a concrete application when he studied the efficacy of phlebotomy (bloodletting). In the eighteenth century and much of the nineteenth, phlebotomy held a position in therapeutics comparable to that of antibiotics today. For inflammatory diseases, such as pneumonia, phlebotomy was the traditional and generally accepted method of treatment. Louis, however, wanted precise quantitative evidence regarding its effectiveness. He wanted to know *how much* benefit resulted from phlebotomy.

With this in mind, Louis studied "pleuropneumonia" (our lobar pneumonia) to settle the specific question, Did bloodletting shorten the course of the disease? In modern terms, his was an entirely retrospective study, based wholly on clinical records.

In this disease, the fairly regular clinical pattern would facilitate measurements. The disease, Louis thought, began with the relatively sudden onset of chills, pain in the chest, and expectoration of rusty sputum. Any earlier symptoms, which we today would call prodromal, he ignored. As his end point he used the start of convalescence, when the patient "began to take some light nourishment; three days at least after the febrile action had ceased."[19] He did not wait for the disappearance of all symptoms.

Within this framework, Louis set himself the question, Did bloodletting shorten the course of pneumonia? His evidence related to the duration of the disease, when subjected to different regimens of bloodletting. Phlebotomy had been used in all cases, so there were no real controls, but the different cases showed varying numbers of bleedings, performed at different points during the disease, and with different amounts of blood removed. All these variables had to be integrated.

From his records, Louis took seventy-eight cases of pneumonia who had been in perfect health when the symptoms first appeared. Of these, twenty-eight died. He tabulated, together with other data, the number of phlebotomies, the day of the illness on which each was performed, and the amount of blood removed. Then he correlated these findings with the duration of the disease, as defined above. The tabulations also took account of data from the patients who died.

From his analysis he concluded that venesection (phlebotomy or bloodletting) did indeed affect the course of pneumonia, but much less than usually asserted. Bloodletting did not relieve pain, nor affect the character of the sputum, nor arrest the disease at once. But if carried out within the first four days after onset of symptoms, phlebotomy could shorten the total duration of the disease by four or five days. However, if performed after the first four days of the disease, the procedure did not affect the total duration. Louis concluded that phlebotomy did have value, or in his words, "a happy effect on the progress of pneumonitis," but he emphasized that this effect was much less than commonly believed (ibid., p. 48).

In this same monograph, Louis applied his method to two other inflammatory diseases, erysipelas and severe tonsillitis (angina tonsillaris), and he also studied the effectiveness of antimony and of vesication as remedies. His results, however, were considerably less definite, and discussion here would not be illuminating. As a statistician, in the modern sense, Louis had grave shortcomings.[20]

DISSEMINATING LOUIS'S IDEAS: JAMES JACKSON

Of the reactions that Louis's method induced among American physicians, the most vivid, perhaps, were those of James Jackson, Sr. (1777–1864). His son had been a student of Louis and had transmitted to his father much that he had learned in Paris. Tragically, at the threshold of a brilliant career, the young man died shortly after his return to Boston. The father, as if to enshrine his son's memory, promoted as best he could some of the new ideas from Paris.

For the translation of Louis's work on bloodletting, Jackson wrote a detailed preface, explaining the numerical method for the benefit of American readers. The need for this we see when Jackson commented, incidentally, "To many of our readers M. Louis is not yet known."[21] This was in 1836, when in this country only leading practitioners were aware of European developments. Only gradually was this awareness heightened by the numerous American students who, after studying in Paris, returned to this country to practice.[22]

Improved therapeutics, the main concern of practitioners, would require increased knowledge of disease, that is, its natural history. Jackson hoped that Louis, "or men like him," would study the effect of remedies in the same way that they carried out their "pathological researches." He predicted that within fifty years the "art of healing will be grounded on many exact rules, which we and our predecessors have not known." These rules must not be deduced from "grand principles" of physiology or pathology (i.e., not from broad and speculative general principles). Instead, the new effective rules "must be deduced from the aggregate of careful, faithful observations of individual facts, made by men of enlightened minds."[23]

From his own cases, Jackson had tried to determine the effectiveness of bloodletting in pneumonia, but his findings, described in an appendix to Louis's book, were quite inconclusive. However, he thought that enough data, from enough cases, would solve the problems. Ten hospitals, he said, "under the care of honest physicians, may settle the questions discussed in this work within five years, so that our posterity will not for ages be able to make any material correction in the answers."

Then he continued to a final sentence that implies an entire philosophy of science. "Seasons and epidemics will vary no doubt; but the general laws will be found the same, and little else will remain for future ages than to settle the allowance to be made for disturbing forces" (ibid., p. 171). Such was the touching faith in facts, patiently and accurately collected, and free from the taint of "hypothesis."

INCREASED APPEAL OF HOMEOPATHY

In the 1830s, Samuel Jackson insisted that medicine was actually a "demonstrative" science, although less exact than physics or chemistry. At the same time, he lamented that medical practice was so "uncertain." Physicians, he said, were relying not on science but on experience. If medicine were to improve and lose the taint of a mere "prescriptive" art, it would need a better application of the "positive" method that characterized science.

Jackson's disquiet was indeed well founded. The proprietary medical schools had debased medical education and were turning out vast numbers of practicing physicians, many of whom were thoroughly ignorant of science. At the same time, sects, especially homeopathy, were becoming stronger.[24] Regular physicians as a class did not have much better therapeutic results than did these sectarians. Moreover, the harsh therapeutic regimen of the regular physicians, usually called heroic therapy, contrasted with the much milder regimen of the sectarians. By the 1840s the American medical profession was experiencing not only a diminished public confidence but also doubts within itself.

As a further difficulty, an economic stringency was affecting regular physicians, due in part to competition from homeopaths and other sectarians, in part to the oversupply of regular practitioners. Economic hardship among physicians was a major factor leading to the formation of the American Medical Association (AMA) in 1847.[25] The self-serving claims that the AMA came into being primarily to raise the level of medical education is only a very partial truth. Economic problems intensified the resentment of regular physicians against homeopaths.

Some prominent regular physicians were questioning the value of traditional therapy and were inclining to a greater trust in nature. Jacob Bigelow's essay on self-limited diseases and Nathan Smith's monograph on typhous fever stimulated a greater reliance on nature. John Harley Warner discussed the increased therapeutic skepticism and the diminished use of harsh remedies in the 1830s and 1840s.[26]

In the rebellion against excessive therapy, a high point occurred in 1860, when Oliver Wendell Holmes published his famous declaration: "I firmly believe that if the whole materia medica, *as now used,* could be sunk to the bottom of the sea, it would be all the better for mankind,—and all the worse for the fishes."[27] This widely quoted statement, however, represented the views of only a part of the profession.

Several different groups were sorting themselves out in the medical profession. We can distinguish, among others, a forward-looking medical elite; a well-trained but conservative and traditionally oriented group; and a broad range of poorly trained practitioners.

Disputes about therapy should be viewed on a larger canvas. They related to the traditional distinction between the science and the art of medicine—between the theory and the practice. Supposedly, practice rested on science, which justified therapeutic procedures. Running parallel to orthodox medicine, homeopathic practice also had an extensive theoretical justification. Oliver Wendell Holmes, in his brilliant essay of 1842, thoroughly demolished the theoretical pretensions of homeopathy.[28]

According to logic, the sect should have withered away, whereas actually it flourished more than ever. Holmes's essay apparently made a greater impression on future historians than it did on the contemporary world. Homeopathy appealed to the general public, for whom only the therapeutic result counted, not the theory behind it.

The difficulties were distressing to well-educated physicians who, despite the empiricism of most medical practice, continued to regard medicine as a science. The increased public confidence in homeopathy was a bitter pill for regular practitioners. In 1846 the situation was much exacerbated.

SIR JOHN FORBES'S CALL FOR CONTROLLED EXPERIMENTS

John Forbes (1784–1861), knighted in 1853, was one of the leading British physicians of his generation. He translated the works of Laennec and Auenbrugger into English (in 1821 and 1824, respectively) and brought auscultation and percussion to the attention of the British medical profession. With two collaborators, he edited the massive *Cyclopedia of Practical Medicine,* completed in 1835, a work frequently cited by American authors. Forbes also edited the influential *British and Foreign Medical Review,* which became the leading medical journal in Great Britain.[29]

This journal generally ignored publications on homeopathy. In 1845, however, because of several recent books, Forbes felt he had to discuss the subject and did so in a long review essay. This, appearing originally in Forbes's journal in January 1846, was quickly reprinted in pamphlet form in Philadelphia by two separate publishers.[30] The paper had a considerable role in shaping the concept of scientific medicine in the United States.

Forbes's essay directly stimulated Elisha Bartlett to write a re-buttal, which became an American treatise on scientific method. Before discussing this I will indicate Forbes's main points.

He first examined the theory of homeopathy, as enunciated by Samuel Hahnemann. However, while blasting its theoretical absurdity, Forbes carefully distinguished between (alleged) thera-peutic results and the explanatory theory behind them. The effec-tiveness of the remedies was regarded as a matter of recorded experience, as allegedly observed fact. Evidence had been offered. It had to be evaluated.

Hahnemann himself had raised the crucial issue half a century before. He declared, it is wrong to ask, What effect *can* 1/100,000th of a grain of belladonna have? The proper question is, rather, What effect *does* 1/100,000th of a grain of belladonna have?[31] Forbes, in his exposition, did not mention this specific query of Hahnemann, but he did encompass its spirit—if therapeutic success was estab-lished, any theoretical absurdity did not negate the fact. At issue were the questions, Was the therapy successful? Did it have any effect? And then there is the further question, How do you know? The question whether homeopathic theory (i.e., its explanations) was true represents a totally different problem. First you must establish your "facts."

For much of his data, Forbes studied the reports of a homeo-pathic hospital in Vienna. Under homeopathic treatment, the mild cases recovered as well as they would have under allopathy, while severe diseases would kill "a considerable proportion" under either therapy.[32] This, however, did not at all imply that homeopathy had "power" over diseases or that homeopathy was "true." Such inferences Forbes utterly rejected. On the other hand, there was no positive evidence that the homeopathic practice was totally "powerless" in treating disease.

The only way to reach a decision would involve an experiment "of a comparative kind, on a large scale, of *its* [homeopathy's] powers, on the one hand, and of *nature's* powers, on the other." Only such an experiment—which we would call controlled—could show whether homeopathy cured better than unaided nature, and whether homeopathic treatment was any better than no treatment at all (ibid., p. 251). While Forbes believed that the supposed benefits of homeopathy derived from the healing power of nature, proof could come only from a properly controlled experiment.

Even the prospect of such a procedure, however, would also cast doubt on the alleged benefits of orthodox therapeutics. Medical tradition had inculcated the belief that nature was inadequate to cure disease (at least, severe disease), but that "art was adequate." These views "have been almost universally received as axioms, without investigation" (p. 253). Forbes, however, wanted investigation. He was emphasizing that a large proportion of the cases treated by allopathic physicians were cured by nature.

He thus raised the question whether, by exalting the powers of nature in reference to homeopathic claims, he might not "at the same time, [be] laying bare the nakedness of our own cherished allopathy?" (p. 253). The answer was clear. "It would, doubtless, be going far beyond the truth to assert, that there is no certainty in medical therapeutics, and that the whole practice of medicine . . . is a system of traditionary routine and conventionalism, haphazard and guesswork; but it is not going beyond the truth to assert, that *much* of it is so" (p. 260).

Forbes told an amusing story of his own earlier dispensary practice, when a little girl was reporting her progress. She felt much better "since Friday." When he asked her what happened on Friday, the child replied, "Please, sir, my medicine was done" (p. 248).

Homeopathy, Forbes believed, had brought into focus the defects of current medical practice. At the same time, he repeatedly stressed the fallacy of post hoc propter hoc reasoning. In so doing, he was really accusing regular physicians of the same logical defects and methodological faults that these orthodox practitioners leveled against homeopaths. He was saying, in essence, it is not enough to count and measure, as Louis had recommended. Scientific medicine required therapeutic experiments that were better controlled. For Forbes, the claims of the homeopaths regarding therapeutic success had no logical force, but the claims of the allopaths were also flawed.

ELISHA BARTLETT'S DEFENSE OF REGULAR MEDICINE

A vigorous denunciation of Forbes's ideas came from Elisha Bartlett, whom William Osler called "a Rhode Island Philosopher."[33] We have met Bartlett earlier, in the discussion of typhoid fever. He received his M.D. degree in 1826 and then studied for a year in Europe, mostly in Paris. On his return to the United States, he practiced in Lowell, Massachusetts, where he also served two terms as mayor. Much of his professional life was that of a peripatetic professor, who wrote prolifically and taught a range of subjects in a number of different medical schools.

His reply to Forbes tried to answer the latter's criticisms but did not grasp their essential features.[34] Bartlett insisted that medicine had "legitimate claims" to the respect of mankind (ibid., p. 11). To establish this, he started by praising the great achievements of medical science (that is, of the individual medical sciences). First he noted the progress in anatomy (including microscopy, embryology, and comparative anatomy) and in physiology, which had ascertained the functions "of nearly all the organs and tissues of the human body" (p. 14). These branches, he said, had reached a "degree of completeness" quite comparable to the natural sciences. He implied that since these latter enjoyed public confidence, medicine should too.

Into another "department" of medical science he placed pathology and therapeutics, which dealt with "the phenomena of disease, and of the means of preventing, mitigating, and removing disease" (p. 17). He focused on our knowledge of pneumonia, in which morbid anatomy, clinical symptoms, and physical signs had been well studied, along with its clinical course and variations in severity. He did, however, admit the obscurity regarding the causes and said we must seek "the circumstances and conditions which seem to favor the production of disease" (p. 27). With such a total accumulation of knowledge, the science of medicine did not in any way deserve "the charges of incompleteness and uncertainty which have been laid at its door" (p. 28).

Medical practice had been indicted as haphazard, a matter of guesswork and conjecture. To disprove this, Bartlett examined in some detail the studies on therapy that Louis and Grisolle had carried out, with special reference to bloodletting. Relying on their findings, Bartlett concluded that "the efficacy of bloodletting in the treatment of pneumonia, is not an error and a delusion; it has its foundation in nature and in truth . . . clear, intelligible, philosophical demonstration" (p. 42).

Bartlett distinguished the mild cases that would get well independent of medical treatment from another group that would inevitably die regardless of medical art. However, in an intermediate group the outcome would depend on treatment. In such cases, bloodletting, he declared, had a "proven control over disease when properly used." And, he added dogmatically, *"it is impossible to doubt"* that it will save the life of the patient *"when properly and promptly applied."* It would, he said, "be utterly illogical and preposterous to doubt this" (pp. 53–54). He had complete confidence that Louis's statistics scientifically proved the validity of medical art.

Bartlett's mind had no room for doubt that medical art did have "power" over pneumonia. And this "proven" success of art in pneumonia seemed to carry over into medical therapy in general. Apparently he could not see a need for additional controls, whether in pneumonia or other diseases.

Bartlett's intended refutation of Forbes relied on the effectiveness of bloodletting in pneumonia. This was "scientifically" demonstrated, according to his concepts of science. He then contrasted the certainty of medicine with the claims of homeopathy, and in so doing he showed how little he understood what Forbes was really trying to do. Homeopaths had not presented any rigorous data to show the efficacy of their system, and their published reports did not "prove" anything. Forbes had already forcefully maintained this, but also insisted that theoretical falsity did not automatically eliminate therapeutic claims. He wanted fully controlled therapeutic trials, including what we would call placebo controls. Homeopaths had never presented such evidence, but then, neither had orthodox medicine.

To determine the value of different remedies, claimed Bartlett, "requires a more thorough and exact knowledge of disease, a longer continued, more extensive, and more assiduous observation at the bedside, sounder judgment . . . a nicer analysis, a more rigorous and inflexible logic, than are necessary to attain any other end in the science." Homeopathy, he said, had never, "on a scale of sufficient magnitude . . . complied with the conditions which are absolutely necessary in order to ascertain the actual and comparative efficacy of its methods of treating disease" (p. 80).

True enough. Yet Forbes had said the very same thing in a different way and in addition wanted greater experimental precision whereby the healing power of nature, by itself, could be identified. In Forbes's view, regular medicine was no more rigorous than homeopathy. Bartlett, who furnished no original evidence of his own, believed that Louis's data had satisfied all possible logical requirements.

Both Forbes and Bartlett were dealing with the reliability of medical science and its methodology. Bartlett, however, was also concerned with the even more basic questions, What *is* medical science? What is its inner or "real" nature?

On this subject, Bartlett's monograph of 1848 expressed his earlier views already stated in 1844 in his well-known book *An Essay on the Philosophy of Medical Science.*[35] This work, however, elaborated on a still earlier and little known published lecture of 1841, given when he assumed the chair of the theory and practice of medicine at Transylvania University. *An Introductory Lecture on the Objects and Nature of Medical Science* presented his ideas to an unsophisticated audience.[36]

Bartlett explained the nature of medical science: its subject matter was unique—the natural history of disease and the ways of curing it—but its methodology was the same as in other and more exact sciences, such as physics and chemistry. Medical science, he declared, investigates all the phenomena of morbid action and relates them to each other and to their causes as well as to therapeutic agents. But its subject matter concerns what is actually observed. Repeatedly, he made the point that medical science deals with "*actual, appreciable* phenomena of morbid action" (ibid., p. 6), that is, data furnished by direct sensory observation.

Earlier writers, he said, had erred greatly when, instead of restricting themselves to the study of phenomena, they indulged in metaphysical speculation. They were seeking the "*ultimate* and *essential nature*" of disease, which was not ascertainable by the senses (p. 7). It was important to make observations, not to speculate about them.

Once these phenomena were ascertained, they had to be analyzed, arranged, and classified, "according to their intimate and obvious relations." This had clear reference to Louis's method of arranging data in tabular form, with the expectation that "obvious relations" would emerge and yield "general facts" or "laws." Such analysis would lead to "the generalization of phenomena." A "general fact"—a generalization from multiple instances—would be a "law" of that particular science. A law, then, is "the expression of a universal fact" (p. 8).

Bartlett gave several examples of such laws, drawn from the data of morbid anatomy. Thus, according to his views, phthisis (tuberculosis) was the deposition of "an extraneous, morbid matter," with certain physical and chemical properties to which we gave the name *tubercle* (p. 14). Another law declared that the tubercle manifested a strong predilection for the apex of the lungs. Another, that in phthisis the morbid process began about two-thirds of the time in the left lung (p. 11). These he considered to be laws of pathology, arrived at through observation and generalization.

When compared with the physical sciences, medical science suffered because the means of observation were so imperfect. Medical phenomena were fugitive and complex, and the relationships they exhibited to each other and to their causes were subtle and inscrutable (p. 9). In medicine, knowledge was approximate only; quite different, he thought, from the laws of the physical sciences.

When, however, phenomena were considered in large aggregates, a much greater accuracy resulted. Bartlett spoke of the "science of vital statistics" (dealing, for example, with births and deaths). The "same process," he thought, might be applied to the phenomena of diseases and thus lead to actual predictions. We must realize that the work of Jules Gavarret on medical statistics, which had such an eventual impact on medicine, had been published only in 1840.[37]

What about theory? It was natural, said Bartlett, that the mind should not be fully satisfied with observations alone. We would want to know the agencies by which these "recondite processes, these phenomena are brought about. We ask for the secret and invisible chain which somehow runs through and binds them together. We demand to know the *how* and the *why* of these facts." The answer would come by way of "theory and hypothesis." He claimed not to object to theory or hypothesis in science. They were "legitimate aids in our search after truth," but they must be kept in their "proper places," which were "very humble and subordinate ones."[38]

Theories that attempted to explain and interpret phenomena were not themselves phenomena (i.e., not directly observable) but only assumptions—speculations. Science, however, "consists in the actual phenomena and their relations—and not in the hypothetical interpretation." Phenomena and their relations were regarded as matters of direct observation and formed the true object of science. They did not depend on theory but were "absolutely independent" of it (ibid., pp. 12–13).

In this essay, Bartlett presented a coherent view of the nature of medical science. He insisted on the primacy of observed phenomena, while theory, interpretation, and explanation held an entirely subordinate place. "Phenomena" and their "relationships" were the proper domain of science. Any theoretical elaboration could have only a limited explanatory role, at best only probable. After allowing for differences in nomenclature, we can sympathize with these views.

Three years later, when Bartlett published his text on the philosophy of medicine, there had been a substantial change. He had become quite rigid and dogmatic in his thinking, and these qualities he coupled with unseemly vituperation and arrogance. Moreover, he used a different phraseology, which impaired cogency and exposed him to serious criticism.

In his new book, science consisted only of "ascertained facts, or phenomena, or events; with their relations to other facts, or phenomena, or events; the whole classified and arranged."[39] Repeatedly, he dismissed the frequently suggested view that, in science, observation supplied only the raw material, which would then be elaborated by a process of reasoning. Instead, he insisted, facts and relations *were* the science, the whole science, and needed no "superadded reasonings or inductions" (ibid., pp. 73, 74).

He was embracing an uncompromising empiricism, wherein knowledge depended only on observation of objective "facts." Indeed, he had become almost violent in rejecting the place of reasoning in science. There was no need for "the *inductive or reasoning process separate from the facts and their relations*" (p. 69). Unfortunately, Bartlett failed to see the infinite complexity of so-called facts and their interconnections (or "relationships"). He considered them in isolation, like the contents of little match boxes that could be closed up, and then stacked and arranged.[40]

FLAWS IN BARTLETT'S CONCEPTS

Bartlett coupled together the terms *facts* and *relationships* and regarded them as the only proper components of science. Both components, he thought, derived from observation. This, of course, is egregious error. A relationship is not observed—it is inferred. It represents an activity of reason leading to a conclusion, namely, that a connection of some sort exists between particular observations. David Hume had already made all this abundantly clear in the eighteenth century.

By explicitly rejecting the reasoning process from medical science, Bartlett thought he was eliminating the hated "rationalism," which he had so despised in Cullen and Rush. He was proud that medicine, in his new formulation, would now be an entirely empirical science, free of rationalism. When, however, he called relationships a matter of observation, his edifice crumbled. What he claimed he had driven out by the door, immediately came back through the window.

This became apparent in his discussion of "general facts," which he equated with "law." To find such a general fact, he could point to a number of individual instances. We may take as examples the autopsy findings in tuberculosis. (We realize, of course, that Bartlett made few investigations of his own but was relying on the data of Louis.) These autopsy findings—facts—were highly complex, but they could be analyzed into simpler components. Through analysis and subsequent arrangement into tables, facts could be laid out like fish on a slab. Then, from many different instances, certain features would, he thought, stand out as similar one to another.

What happened was a process of abstraction, whereby from highly complex aggregates of observation the pathologist noted certain similarities and selected particular features, which he placed in a separate class. By so doing, he indicated a relation between certain observed features.

With this in mind, we can examine some "laws" that Bartlett asserted for phthisis: a peculiar kind of "morbid matter," deposited in the lungs, affected the left more often than the right, and with a special predilection for the apex. These were "general facts," which supposedly were made manifest by observation alone, without any "reasoning."

Bartlett did not appreciate the basic difference between an observation, recorded as datum of experience, and a generalization. The latter is a *conclusion,* which jumps from some instances of a phenomenon, already observed, to all instances that may occur in the future and have not yet been observed. This passage from some to all is the inductive leap that creates the generalization. It is very different from a description of something past, which does not involve any jump.

The description of a past observation comprises a historical fact. An example would be, The first ten cases of phthisis examined showed the left lung more severely involved than the right. As a historical datum, this would be adequately descriptive. If we wanted to generalize, we might say, Phthisis usually starts in the left lung. This would then be a "law." We would be passing from some instances, observed in the past, to all instances that might occur in the future. Bartlett did not distinguish between description of historical events and induction leading to generalization.

If the observations (historical facts) were noted carefully and accurately, the inductive leap would land on reasonably firm ground. If, however, the original observations were careless, they would be "false facts," and any inductive leap based upon them would land in a quagmire. Whoever makes a generalization leaves the assured ground of observation for an uncertain prediction of the future. Such an implicit prediction was the essence of Bartlett's

scientific or "general" fact. This contrasted sharply with the historical fact recorded in observations, which by themselves carried no
prediction.

By a rather idiosyncratic use of language, Bartlett applied the
term *relationship* to cover all the activities that earlier writers had
assigned to reason. He ignored the rational aspects of making
judgments and comparisons, of identifying similarities and differences. These features he called "relationships," and thought we
became aware of them through empirical observation.

His motivation, I believe, was simple. Bartlett had a passionate
hatred of "system," that is, the organization of knowledge into a
unified whole, where every part had a logical connection with every
other part. In eighteenth-century medical systems, a great deal of
inference might rest on a slender basis of actual observation. This
was especially the case with therapy, where inference alone might
yield procedures with negligible basis in actual experience. Bartlett, concerned with treatment rather than theory, wanted therapy
to rest on a firm foundation of observations, not on reasoning or
hypothesis. Therapeutics, he claimed, could not be deduced from
the principles of pathology. Each branch of medical science must
rest on its own observations.

As a philosopher, Bartlett was only third rate, and his failings
were apparent to his contemporaries. Robley Dunglison (1798–
1869), for example, condemned "the disposition . . . to narrow down
the science of medicine to the mere observation of facts," and he
explicitly considered *The Philosophy of Medical Science* guilty of
this fault. John Forbes, when reviewing the book, praised Bartlett's
advocacy of "careful and accurate observation of the phenomena
of disease, as the only source of real improvements in medical
practice." But he also emphasized at length the importance of
hypothesis, which Bartlett had rejected.[41]

Alfred Stillé also provided relevant comments on relationships
and on what I call the inductive leap. His own pathology text of 1848
included an essay entitled "Medical Truth. Its Nature, Sources, and
Means of Attainment."[42] In this he emphasized that mere industry
in collecting data was not enough. All wits were not on a level.
There was, instead, a genius, a power of penetrating into things
and of perceiving essential differences. He pointed to major figures

in medicine as men who "saw relations amongst the phenomena of disease, which were invisible to less gifted men, and, having seen them by virtue of their genius, they did not stop there, and build up a theory upon them . . . but immediately applied themselves to discover *whether they had seen correctly;* they tested their inspirations by observation and experiment" (ibid., pp. 46–47).

This insight into relationships represents the aha reaction, with the added virtue of seeking empirical demonstration of that insight. These were essential features of science that Bartlett had missed. Stillé, however, fully grasped the essence of the scientific method. The relationships between phenomena, which Bartlett claimed were identified through observations alone, were actually perceived through insight, or genius. This meant an operation of the mind, an activity that was part of reason. Some persons had this genius, others did not.

HYPOTHESIS AND VERIFICATION

Although Bartlett claimed that medical science followed the methods of the more exact sciences, he had no real awareness of the methodology in these sciences. This we see vividly with certain events of 1846. Bartlett condemned all explanations in science that invoked hypotheses to clarify phenomena. Every attempt "to refer these phenomena to certain unknown and assumed conditions for the purpose of rendering them rational, has been to hinder the progress and improvement of the science."[43]

At the very time he was writing these words, events in astronomy were proving him utterly mistaken. One of the long-troublesome problems in that science had been the irregularities in the orbit of the planet Uranus. Two astronomers, John C. Adams and U. J. J. Le Verrier, one British and one French, calculated independently that the anomalous movements could be explained by assuming the existence of another planet. So sound were the calculations that in 1846 a relatively brief search sufficed to locate in the sky the postulated body, now called Neptune. Scientists facing confusing observations rendered them orderly and rational—explained them—by introducing certain hypothetical conditions. This was exactly what Bartlett condemned. The great divergence was that the astronomers verified their assumptions in experience.

EVALUATION OF BARTLETT'S WORK

Bartlett's formulation of scientific medicine, although widely quoted by historians, actually had little contemporary influence. Boerhaave and Cullen had already insisted that medical science must rest on observation, and that observations should be elaborated by reason. Bartlett followed Louis in wanting observations to be abundant, precise, detailed, and adequately documented. But he did not understand the role of hypothetical reasoning.

Bartlett himself was a clinician, and not in any sense an investigator. He kept referring to "medical science," as if medicine comprised one unified discipline that he could compare to the exact sciences. Actually, the individual medical sciences—anatomy, physiology, chemistry, and pathology—did bear comparison with the physical sciences in many ways, despite the great differences in precision. The *practice* of medicine, however, was quite different from medical sciences. Practice was essentially empirical, in its pejorative sense. To make clinical medicine (practical medicine) scientific, Louis wanted to introduce an improved methodology, involving some degree of quantitation and rudimentary controls, all epitomized as the "numerical method." Bartlett wanted to help this innovation but did not know how.

Earlier I mentioned three aspects of medical science: concepts, method, and technology. Bartlett did not appreciate the importance of new conceptual and technological advances, nor of experiment based on hypothesis. The real illumination that Forbes provided did not penetrate to Bartlett. Trying to reform practical medicine by juggling terms that he did not fully understand was merely a quixotic gesture. Medical practice might eventually become scientific, but only after a prolonged development of concepts, methods, and technology. Only then would science exert some concrete influence on practice. Bartlett would be left hopelessly behind, one of the major failures of the 1840s.

9

Medicine as Art and Science, 1850–1912

TODAY, AT THE END OF TWENTIETH CENTURY, WE ARE acutely aware that socioeconomic, cultural, and political factors affect all aspects of medicine. In the first half of the nineteenth century the same influences were also operative, but their effects were far less obvious. After midcentury, however, the cultural changes that influenced medicine were becoming more and more intrusive. We may, perhaps, regard this second half of the century as an era of special conflicts.

After the Civil War there was massive expansion on all fronts. Of particular relevance were industrialization, immigration, the growth and transformation of capitalism, economic uncertainty, the increasing self-consciousness of labor, and the growth of economic (and later, of political) imperialism. These represent but a few of the influences—and resulting conflicts—that affected medicine.

Another significant feature was the expansion of science and its practical effects on everyday life.[1] More and more the public became aware of science as something affecting both intellectual attitudes and practical living. Science and things scientific were acquiring a status that gradually permeated all levels of society.

Science, of course, has innumerable facets, whose relations to medicine may be studied on several levels. If we select a few particular features and trace them through half a century, we may achieve a synoptic view of medical transformations and some of the dynamics involved.

In the overall intellectual and social environment I will focus on three aspects. One I call elitism, with its overtones of trade unionism. The formation of special groups—associations, colleges, and societies are the chief designations—has been a powerful determinant in medical development. A second area for study concerns the division of medicine into its theoretical and practical aspects, later expressed by the phrase, the science and the art of medicine. This aspect, in turn, involves the subject of medical education. My third area for analysis deals with those components of medical science that I have already identified as conceptual, technological, and methodological.

ELITISM AND THE FORMATION OF THE AMERICAN MEDICAL ASSOCIATION

The drives toward elitism were in part ideological, in part economic. A splendid example is the formation of the American Medical Association (AMA), in 1847.[2] The competition from homeopaths and other sects was having severe economic repercussions and also was affecting the pride of well-trained physicians. At the preliminary convention of 1846, committees were formed to report on problems and to propose remedies. The report of the Committee on Ethics revealed some of the latent motives.

One complaint declared that the community did not hold physicians in proper esteem. They should, said the report, be tendered the same respect and consideration accorded to lawyers and clergymen. "Truly learned" physicians should not be regarded in the same light as "ignorant pretenders" nor should their practice be lumped together with the "crooked devices and low arts" of "interloping empirics."[3]

Various comments emphasized the proper methodology of science, as exemplified by the medical profession. Physicians were "enjoined . . . not to advance any statement unsupported by positive facts, nor to hazard an opinion or hypothesis that is not the result of deliberate inquiry" (ibid. p. 88). This, of course, was the opposite of quackery, but the very exhortation suggests a considerable deficiency in this regard among regular physicians.

Physicians should set themselves apart, said the report. As

"trustees of science . . . physicians should use unceasing vigilance to prevent the introduction into their body of those who have not been prepared by suitably preparatory moral and intellectual training" (p. 90). Human life should "not be endangered by the incompetency of presumptious pretenders." All this was aimed at homeopaths and other sectarians. The physician, with his superior knowledge, must not give the "slightest countenance," still less support, to any such "empirical imposture" (p. 87).

The AMA code of ethics strictly forbade any consultation with homeopaths or other irregular practitioners. The AMA had set itself up as an elite group that wanted to preseve its ideological purity, to give at least lip service to the ideals of education, and incidentally to promote its own economic security. This prohibition against consulting with sectarians would profoundly (although indirectly) affect the development of modern scientific medicine. The paths lay through the thickets of elitism.

The AMA was not able to bring its own house into good order. The organization could take a united stand against homeopaths but could do little to protect the public against physicians who were poorly trained and incompetent.[4] Various efforts failed, for a variety of reasons. Within the medical profession, one elite subgroup, the American Academy of Medicine, protested strongly against this failure.[5] This organization, founded in 1876, wanted to promote especially high educational standards for entrance into medical schools. Besides demanding real improvement in education, the academy wanted to promote sound critical judgment and the ability to reason and evaluate evidence.[6] In a sense this was trying to make actual the ideals that the AMA had hinted at thirty years before, at a time when such goals were rather visionary.

Specialization in medicine gave an enormous impetus to the formation of elite societies; each specialty group wanted to establish an identity, promote scientific standards, and make progress in scientific achievements. At the same time, the group could, in good guild fashion, promote the welfare of its members against less qualified competitors. The groups, whether called societies or associations, were national in scope, not merely local.

Ophthalmologists and otologists formed such speciality societies in 1864 and 1866, respectively. Psychiatrists, dermatologists, gynecologists, and laryngologists created similar organizations between 1875 and 1879. In 1880 the American Surgical Association was formed. Clearly, it was only a matter of time before leaders in internal medicine would also establish their own association. In fact, this took place in 1885, but against a quite remarkable background.

MEDICAL ETHICS, SO-CALLED, AND THE AMERICAN ASSOCIATION OF PHYSICIANS

For our purposes, the most important elite organization of the era was the American Association of Physicians (AAP), founded in 1885.[7] Its origin was precipitated by a dispute over medical ethics, so-called, a dispute that revealed the intense interpenetration of social, economic, and scientific factors.

As we have seen, the AMA at its formation in 1847 imposed an "ethical" ban on consultations between physicians and homeopaths. By 1876 enlightened physicians realized that this prohibition did not work, and the president of the AMA in that year pointed out that modifications would be necessary. Although the AMA paid no heed, the State Medical Society of New York, in 1882, drew up a new ethical code. This eliminated references to doctrinal orthodoxy and permitted open consultation between legally qualified practitioners. Since in New York homeopaths had the same legal rights as regular physicians, consultations between the two groups would not violate ethical guidelines. This new code was adopted only after much intricate political infighting, of a very unsavory kind.

By adopting the new code, the New York State Society cut itself off from the AMA and went on its own independent way. Meanwhile, New York adherents of the AMA code formed a new state association, which maintained ties with the AMA. The resulting schism in New York, with two conflicting medical societies, lasted until 1906.

Meanwhile, in 1884, the AMA planned to host a meeting of the International Congress of Medicine, to be held in Washington, D.C., in 1887. A committee was appointed to make appropriate arrangements and draw up a program. The committee, headed by John S. Billings, enlisted outstanding American participants and presented its report to the annual meeting of the AMA at the end of April 1885.

Then there occurred an episode exceedingly disgraceful to the AMA. Many of the names Billings proposed were members of the New York State Society, which had embraced the new code, anathema to AMA orthodoxy. The AMA formally rejected the report because it gave prominent positions to new-code adherents. To scuttle the report, parliamentary maneuvers were dressed up in plausible excuses. For example, it was claimed that the various officers and chairman originally appointed did not provide a fair geographical distribution of physicians. By making a different geographical distribution, the old hard-liners could eliminate new-code adherents from the program.

The AMA appointed a new committee to draw up a different list of major participants. There resulted a tremendous outcry from leading physicians all over the country, including Samuel Gross, S. Weir Mitchell, William Osler, Oliver Wendell Holmes, Reginald Fitz, William Pepper, and Francis Minot, to name but a few. By September 1885, the storm of protests forced the new committee to retreat from its rigid stand and to repair the damage as best it could. However, only a few of the more distinguished American physicians consented to appear on the final program.

Meanwhile, in October 1885, only a few months after the high-handed AMA actions, definite plans were being made to establish the American Association of Physicians. Organization proceeded promptly, and the first meeting was held in 1886, with Francis Delafield as its president.

His inaugural address is quite unintelligible unless we understand the stormy actions of the previous year. He declared, "We are an association in which there will be no medical politics and no medical ethics; an association in which no one will care who are the officers and who are not; in which we will not ask what part of the country a man comes from, but whether he has done good work and will do more." This was a completely explicit condemnation of the earlier AMA action.

The unequivocal statement of motives clearly explains why the AAP was established at that particular time. However, had it not been founded 1885–86, it inevitably would have come into being at some other time. It expressed the trend to specialization and the formation of elite societies to promote their aims. Fortunately, the aims of the AAP were entirely scientific and unselfish. It was a truly prestigious organization, elitism at its best, and it turned its back on medical politics that masqueraded as ethics.

Membership in the AAP, which included pathologists as well as internists, represented the very top layer of American medicine. While its members made important contributions to clinical medicine, more relevant for our purpose was the analysis of scientific medicine that we find in a few scattered papers. These belong in the area I call the methodology of science. This in turn was closely bound up with technological advances. For consideration of the subject, I pass over the clinical considerations and limit myself to some features crucial to pathology.

DEPENDENCE ON MICROSCOPY

At midcentury, cell theory was the great conceptual advance that changed the course of pathology. This concept, however, developed out of technological improvements in microscopy, which gave new insights into the structure of normal tissues and the morbid changes that might affect them. The greatest progress took place in Europe, especially in Germany. At the same time, experimental techniques helped to define fresh problems for study and led to new conceptual advances. The third quarter of the nineteenth century was a very fertile period in European pathology.

In the United States, however, progress was slow. Here, microscopy did play a small part in advancing anatomy and "natural history" but much less in unravelling the problems of pathology.[8] In this field, the gross autopsy continued to play its role in the study of disease and the training of specialists in internal medicine. Experience in postmortem dissections greatly benefited individual physicians and increased their skill in clinical work. So far as concerned academic advancement, physicians with substantial autopsy experience held a distinct advantage over colleagues limited to clinical experience alone. By the 1870s, long experience in the dissecting room was often a stepping-stone to clinical advancement. William Osler was one among many such examples.

Slowly and painfully, microscopy was also beginning to play a part in the care of patients. A few hospitals established positions for a microscopist, who might double in chemistry. In the Philadelphia General Hospital such a post was created in 1866, but only three microscopic examinations were recorded for that year. By 1871 the number had increased to only twenty-one, when William Pepper, Jr. (1843–99) was the "curator." The first official pathologist was James Tyson (1841–1919), appointed in 1871. Tyson later became the leading clinician in Philadelphia and author of an important textbook.[9]

In medical school little attention was paid to microscopy. William H. Welch (1850–1934) graduated in 1875 from the College of Physicians and Surgeons in New York. As a student he acquired a great deal of autopsy experience but wrote to his father, "I understand pretty well the lesions visible to the naked eye, but I know nothing about the microscopical appearances. I am sorry I have not yet been able to study with the microscope, but hope to find opportunity for it some time."[10] After graduation, Welch studied extensively in Germany, and on his return in 1876 he helped support himself by giving private lessons in microscopy.

The passage of ten years made a considerable difference in educational practices. George Dock (1850–1951), who entered medical school at the University of Pennsylvania in 1881, related that he had had sound training in the use of the microscope. After graduation, he studied gross and microscopic pathology in Germany, as well as bacteriology.[11] Yet he, too, was primarily a clinician.

To study pathology, Americans went eagerly to Germany, where specialists were making rapid advances; but on their return, the Americans usually turned back to clinical medicine. However attractive microscopy might be, it was essentially an academic discipline and opportunities for remunerative work were relatively scanty.

Pathology was undergoing specialization, becoming more and more dependent on microscopy. The older ritual, wherein a clinician would become quite adept at gross examinations and spend long periods in the dissecting room to further his education, was growing obsolete. A new era was coming into being, for which microscopy and all that it stood for served as a symbol.

This new era, the climax of nineteenth-century medicine, established different norms for scientific medicine. The components were many. Of those holding special relevance, microscopy was one, chemistry was another, and bacteriology, as discussed in chapter 7, a third.

The microscope, as a research tool, contributed markedly to the advancement of knowledge. But when it began to play a practical role in the care of patients, a new era began. There developed clinical science, on the one hand, and laboratory medicine, on the other. Technology, methodology, and conceptual advances combined to transform the whole notion of scientific medicine.

MEDICINE AS A SCIENCE: JOHN SHAW BILLINGS

Nineteenth-century physicians concerned themselves with the questions, To what degree was medicine a science? and What was the real distinction between the art and the science? In the 1840s, as we have seen, Bartlett expounded one viewpoint, strongly affected by the methodological advances of Louis earlier in the century.

In 1877 John S. Billings, in lectures that profoundly affected the course of American medicine, dealt incidentally with the problem of art versus science in medicine.[12] Billings had been a guiding genius of the Johns Hopkins University, founded in 1876. The associated hospital did not open until 1889, and the medical school, not until 1893. Billings's lectures of 1877 provided a blueprint for an elite medical school, with standards even higher than those expressed by the American Association of Physicians.

Within the preceding ten years, Billings declared, he had examined some 200 essays and lectures "that wanted to prove that Medicine is a science," and each of them weakened rather than strengthened his faith in that proposition. There were sciences in medicine, such as physiology or pathology or therapeutics, but if we combine them "we get, not precisely a Science of Medicine, but the scientific side of medicine; that which deals with causation or prediction as regards disease." This might be considered "the Science of Medicine in opposition or contrast to the Art. Yet the science . . . is not to be studied apart from the art" (ibid., p. 320).

The faculty of Johns Hopkins's new medical school, said Billings, should increase knowledge and fit its students to increase knowledge. A part of the work of a medical school was to teach the practical applications of this new knowledge. Nevertheless, this effort must be "the secondary and not the primary object" (p. 321). Billings in a sense was really intensifying the distinction between the science and the art of medicine, while holding them insepa-rable.

THE RELATION OF SCIENCE AND ART:
WILLIAM DRAPER

In the decade after Billings wrote, medical knowledge increased enormously. By 1888 the medical sciences had not only made vast substantive advances but had also become dependent on special technology that required considerable training to achieve compe-tence. As a result, the relation between medical science and medi-cal practice became quite convoluted. William Draper (1830–1901), a founding member of the AAP and its president in 1888, tried to integrate the science and the art. He presented his views in a truly landmark paper, entitled "On the Relation of Scientific to Practical Medicine."[13] Practical medicine, we recall, meant only medical practice, or clinical medicine.

Draper wanted to get clinical medicine into the domain of medi-cal science. His views were in part traditional. The science and the art of medicine could be differentiated but not practically dissoci-ated. They were interwoven like the warp and the woof. The scien-tist pursued knowledge for the sake of "knowing what is veiled in obscurity." The practitioner (he used the term "artsman," as the one who practiced the art of medicine) "cultivates science for the sake of learning how to do something that needs to be done."

Draper, however, pointed out the special domains of each group. Whereas the pathologist, for example, was concerned with the causation of disease, the practitioner dealt with the "dynamics" of disease, in the study of which he occupied a field of observation "peculiarly his own." Draper did not clarify precisely what he meant by "dynamics," but he did suggest some particular topics for investi-gation—personal idiosyncrasies; correlation of structure and func-tion; reactions to food and medicine; and the relation of disease to heredity, age, sex, occupation, and environment. These would offer scientific opportunities for the practicing physician, "and require essentially the scientific spirit for their successful cultivation."

Two features here call for comment. The topics Draper sug-gested for investigation required careful observation, but they were not dependent on technological expertise. Draper thought that the worker in science and the worker in the art of medicine might often be combined "in a high degree in the same individual," but this was becoming less and less true. In pathology, for example, microscopic examination of tissues was generally beyond the capacity of most clinicians, even those skilled in gross autopsies. The subjects Draper recommended for study did not require special laboratory skills but were well within the scope of older clinicians.

Second, Draper mentioned, but without elaboration, the need for a "scientific spirit." He did not offer any examples or provide any analysis, yet whatever investigations the clinician might carry out must, he thought, be performed according to scientific canons. In the next dozen or so years, other writers did offer extensive comments on what might characterize the scientific spirit.

Medical art, Draper insisted, must assimilate the discoveries in the etiology of disease, in physiology, and in organic chemistry and make them "all contribute to more exact diagnosis and to more rational therapy." While Draper foresaw great progress in the healing art resulting from discoveries in, say, bacteriology, this would come "mainly from the independent and judicious application of new ideas to the study and treatment of diseases by practical physicians at the bedside."

This was an invitation to establish more firmly the discipline of clinical pathology, which had already had a tenuous beginning and which expanded greatly over the next dozen years.[14] Meanwhile, medical art would provide an impetus to science by continually providing new problems to solve. Furthermore, art would also serve to test the "theorems" of science and to check dangerous and premature exuberance. For example, Draper warned that "the doctrine of parasitism," or bacteriology, might be "forging new errors in diagnosis, and beguile us into dangerous paths in therapeutics." This last seems almost a premonition of Koch's great blunder in the treatment of tuberculosis, when he introduced the use of tuberculin as a therapeutic agent.

Draper, at age fifty-five, was the oldest of the founding members of the AAP. He was not personally well versed in the newer technologies, and his suggested research problems link him to the older physicians. Younger members of the AAP were more laboratory minded.

PROGRESS IN CLINICAL SCIENCE

In his broad survey, Draper underestimated the importance that the microscope would have in uniting the science and the art of medicine. This would take place through clinical pathology. From the historical standpoint, the earliest example of this discipline is probably the examination of the urine. Here we find the use of special observations to identify certain phenomena deemed helpful in diagnosis. Medieval writings on uroscopy and the existence of "piosse prophets" need not detain us here; I would note only that many modern studies on urinalysis were published in the nineteenth century. In 1863, for example, there appeared in English a massive volume of 459 pages entitled *A Guide to the Qualitative and Quantitative Analysis of the Urine*, with the subtitle *Designed Especially for the Use of Medical Men.*[15] This, however, should be construed as a compendium of knowledge, rather than a useful practical guide. In 1870 the average practitioner had at best only a nodding acquaintance with chemistry, and he could not even use a microscope. However, he might have learned a few simple manipulative techniques through which he could have detected the presence of albumin or sugar. Such information would certainly have helped him in diagnosis, but on an empirical basis. It was not clinical science.

What Draper had in mind, actually, was the cooperation of science and art to advance total medical knowledge. The work on malaria, beginning in 1880, illustrates splendidly the way microscopic investigations helped to transform pathology (considered as morbid anatomy) into clinical pathology and clinical science.

In 1880 Charles Laveran (1845–1922), a French army surgeon, noted in the blood of malaria patients small bodies that he considered the causal agent, later identified as a plasmodium.[16] His observations were soon confirmed, but the role of the minute bodies remained uncertain. In 1885 George Sternberg (1838–1915), the leading American microbiologist, then in Europe, saw some of the microscopic preparations. On his return to America, he demonstrated the organisms to Welch, at the Johns Hopkins University. Although the hospital and medical school at the new university had not yet opened, Welch had already been appointed professor of pathology and was engaged in research and some teaching.[17]

William Councilman, Welch's assistant in pathology, published in 1887 a confirmatory paper regarding the hematozoa. Osler, still working in Philadelphia, was stimulated by the research coming out of Baltimore. He studied the blood of seventy patients with malaria, and his resulting paper was an important American contribution to the subject.[18]

Osler, not only an outstanding clinician but also a skilled microscopist, directed his expertise to studying the blood rather than the solid tissues. His work on malaria was a research project that applied the technical skills of a scientist to the diagnostic problems of a clinician. In time, the examination of blood to assist the diagnosis of malaria changed from a research project to a routine procedure, performed first by resident physicians, then by medical students, and then by specially trained technicians.

Microscopic examinations of other body fluids, secretions, and excretions became useful in direct proportion of the growth of special laboratories where such work could be done. Furthermore, personnel had to be trained to carry out such examinations. The clinical laboratory emerged as a major factor in the "scientization" of American medicine.

Studies on malaria are merely one example. Further exposition here must proceed along two parallel paths that developed mostly in the last decade of the century. One concerns the expansion of the clinical laboratory and forms a part of the history of hospitals. It also leads to areas concerned with medical education. The other main path has to do with the concept of the scientific spirit and the changes that this notion underwent over the next two decades. Draper, in a time of confusion, had glimpsed both of the paths, and had some idea, however dim, of where they could lead.

THE SLOW GROWTH OF HOSPITAL LABORATORIES

By the 1870s a few of the better hospitals had set aside small areas for laboratory work, but by the 1890s such facilities were still severely inadequate. I will note three major institutions that by the mid-1890s were establishing standards for the rest of the country.

At the Massachusetts General Hospital, the trustees reported in 1893 that laboratory work was being done "partly in a little den fitted up under the front steps and unfit for human occupation; partly in the nurses' rooms connected with the wards; partly at the Medical School, a mile away; partly at the pathological room in the department of outpatients, where the pathologist is now on duty for one morning a week; and partly in a small room . . . ill adapted . . . for the work which has to be done and for which there is no other place."[19] Following this report, the hospital built a special laboratory building, opened in 1896, which contained facilities considered ample for the time. A resident pathologist was appointed, who soon assumed the title of director of the Clinico-Pathological Laboratory.

An event in 1894 was especially important for the history of laboratories. The William Pepper Laboratory of Clinical Medicine was opened, in honor of William Pepper, Sr. (1810–64). The purpose of the building, specified in the deed of gift, was to promote the interests of the patients "by the prosecution of minute clinical studies and original researches." The donor wanted to bring about "improvement in methods of diagnosing and treating the diseases of human beings."[20] Better patient care and medical research were the watchwords.

At the dedication ceremonies of the Pepper Laboratory, Welch gave a thoughtful address.[21] While the pursuit of science, he pointed out, requires adequate facilities, special laboratories for the medical sciences were a phenomenon chiefly of the nineteenth century. He briefly surveyed the way laboratories were established in disciplines like physiology, chemistry, physiological chemistry, pathology, pharmacology, and "hygiene" (the last referring, I believe, principally to bacteriology). Welch noted that scientific methods (meaning techniques) were passing into the hospitals, and diseases were being studied "with the aid of physical and chemical and microscopical methods."

A hospital laboratory examined the material removed from the patient, such as blood, serous fluids, sputum and other secretions, gastric contents, and fragments of tissue taken for diagnosis. In physiology and other medical sciences, the laboratory dealt with problems that might have "apparently no immediate and direct bearing upon practical medicine," even though in the long run there might be great practical utility. The clinical laboratory, however, concerned itself with questions "which bear directly upon the diagnosis and treatment of disease."

In retrospect, we see that the clinical or hospital laboratory would provide a relatively new subject matter for scientific investigation. Technologies of science were becoming "practical," that is, having a direct bearing on medical practice. Such investigation would have not only immediate practical value but could also advance general knowledge, as befits any science.

Despite all these manifest advantages, hospitals were relatively slow in creating such laboratories. In 1896, Henry Hurd, the superintendent of the Johns Hopkins Hospital, made an eloquent plea, which tells us much by indirection.[22] Hospital construction was proceeding rapidly, and he urged that they should all have increased laboratory facilities, which would use the methods of chemistry, microscopy, bacteriology, and pathology. After referring to the new Pepper Laboratory, Hurd mentioned that money had been donated to the Johns Hopkins Hospital for a similar building. He expressed the fervent wish "that equal liberality would make it possible to hope for similar laboratories in connection with every large hospital in the country."

In 1900 an important paper continued the same theme and added some interesting details.[23] The author, C. N. B. Camac, spoke of research laboratories where "large problems were worked on and methods developed for the detection of disease *per vitam.*" The hospital laboratory, the "offspring" of the research laboratory, was a "workshop where the methods planned and perfected in the other laboratories are applied and given a practical test." Camac favored small ward laboratories, which demanded little space and little money. A useful ward laboratory, he estimated, could be set up for about $300, including a microscope, and would cost only $50 to $75 for annual maintenance. Internes would do the work. A larger hospital would need two internes and a bacteriologist, while in charge would be "a microscopist who was also a chemist."

SPECIAL TRAINING FOR ACADEMIC PHYSICIANS

In 1895, ten years after its founding, William Osler was president of the AAP. In his presidential remarks, he summed up the elitist view of clinical science.[24] Noting that the association's original intent had been "the advancement of scientific and practical medicine," he quoted Delafield's remarks that the new society was not concerned with medical politics or medical ethics. Then he quickly surveyed the high points of papers read in the preceding ten years and published in the annual *Transactions*. The contributions, impressive indeed, had certainly fulfilled the aims enunciated at the founding.

The association, he declared, had strongly influenced the study of pathology and clinical medicine, but more men were needed who could devote themselves to such studies. The progress made by medical schools had resulted in a shortage of well-trained men to fill the teaching positions. Accurate and prolonged training was necessary, but the country did not yet understand "the art of training special clinical physicians."

Such men did not develop out of the routine of family practice. "The time has come when able young men should be encouraged to devote themselves to internal medicine as a specialty. Content to labor and wait during the first ten or fifteen yeas of professional life, with pathology as the solid basis of development, such men will pass to the wards through the laboratories thoroughly equipped to study the many problems of clinical medicine."

These remarks represented the pinnacle of elitism, and in one sense Osler was emphasizing the difference between the AAP and the AMA. The repetition of Delafield's scathing words suggest that the medico-political events of 1885 had left deep scars. The academics were being separated from the general practitioners, and the distinction between "town and gown" was becoming more acute. The clinical laboratory and clinical science would play a major part in the social and professional turmoil affecting various contexts of medicine.

COMPLICATIONS IN THE CONCEPT OF SCIENTIFIC MEDICINE

For centuries there had been a fairly clear distinction between the science and the art of medicine. Science furnished concepts, explanations, and generalizations and also tried to expand total general knowledge (expressed in terms often called laws). The art (or practice) of medicine was not concerned with increasing that total body of knowledge but only with the cure of the individual patient. In this process, diagnosis was an important step, for it provided the indications for therapy.

In the past, investigations in medical science had little direct influence on diagnosis and therapeutics. Only in the later nineteenth century did the results of scientific investigation substantially affect practice. After a relatively slow buildup, this influence expanded almost explosively in the 1890s. By this time, medicine was supposedly becoming increasingly scientific. Just what this meant, however, was not entirely clear.

Two distinct components were mentioned as if they were interchangeable. One was the technical demonstration of important factors. The bacillus of tuberculosis could be directly observed, as could the hematozoon of malaria; blood corpuscles could be enumerated; sugar in the urine could be determined quantitatively; and cancer cells could be seen under the microscope. These achievements, the results of science, offered a precision that seemed to eliminate doubt and guesswork. In a flush of enthusiasm, the clinicians who used such technology considered themselves scientific.

Science, however, had a further essential component, epitomized in the phrase "scientific method." Even though in the 1890s this term did not have the rich meaning it enjoys today, it still conveyed the sense of critical analysis and judgment, experimentation, and verification of hypothesis. All this was not yet rigidly schematized, as it tends to be today, but was regarded as a way of approaching problems—a mode of thought that characterized the scientist. This aspect was taking on an increasing importance.

In 1893, A. L. Loomis (1831–95), president of the American Association of Physicians, declared in his presidential remarks that "the final test of a scientific mind is its power of deciding, after any given demonstration, between legitimate conclusions and unfounded inference."[25] Loomis was, so to speak, an old-timer, intellectually nourished in the medicine of the 1870s. He could see the course of future medicine, with its technical precision, but he himself could not meaningfully participate. Instead, he championed a critical attitude, sound reasoning, and logical conclusions drawn from the data.

Of these two separable components of science, one related to technical procedures, the other to critical judgment. One involved precise techniques, the other, habits of thought. Since they both represented methods of science, the term *scientific methods,* by itself, did not distinguish between the two. Confusion resulted.

In 1897 Arthur Tracy Cabot (1852–1912), a surgeon, wrote a fascinating article entitled "Science in Medicine."[26] He was more than twenty years younger than Loomis, and the newer medical procedures had fully colored his educational and intellectual background. In his presentation, he compared the family doctor of fifty years earlier with the new breed of specialist. The former, thought Cabot, practiced the "empiric art." He had cultivated the powers of observation and paid attention to slight physical signs that the "modern physician" would not notice. The latter, however, had his "instruments of precision," including the clinical thermometer, blood counts, and other microscopic examinations. These, said Cabot, provide better guides "to a correct opinion," so that the physician "does not need observation of the lighter straws to see which way the wind is blowing."

Cabot praised research workers, especially in microscopy and bacteriology, who had laid the foundations of "modern" medicine. In America, the growth of laboratories and the "scientific exactitude" that they brought were changing the practice of medicine. The physician who, in a difficult diagnosis, used precise laboratory methods, "demonstrates the supremacy of scientific over empiric medicine." Furthermore, the physician who uses "exact scientific methods in his practice" would exert considerable influence in his community.

Precise data were replacing mere "opinion." We recall that Louis condemned the use of vague terms in situations where more exact data could be obtained. Judgments based on crude observation were regarded as empiricism, while judgments resting on precise determinations and expressing quantitative values supposedly reflected science.

Cabot pointed out that the busy practitioner might not have the time or the ability to perform all the desired tests, but he might be able to find someone "fresh from the laboratories" who could do the work for him. This was especially true in surgery, where, he said, the prudent man needs the assistance of a trained microscopist.

Laboratory work was being recognized as clinically important, but who would do it? Here we can see the difficulty a generation gap could bring. Young practitioners had had the opportunity to acquire skills that the older generation lacked but was just beginning to need. Progress had enhanced the value of microscopy. As laboratories, where such work could be done, became important for hospitals, hospital privileges with easy access to laboratories were important for progressive clinicians. A new status, a new elitism, developed among practitioners who could rely on a hospital laboratory. At the same time, there was a slow movement toward private laboratories, to which any practitioner, hospital-based or not, might have access.

The "trained physician," Cabot believed, must put the devices of science to constant use. He must be well versed in preventive medicine, the isolation of contagious diseases, the "scientific" study of the water supply and sewage disposal, and other aspects of public health. Not until these various duties had been met could a man "claim to be a scientific practitioner." Cabot pointed to vast knowledge to be mastered, as well as the tools of precision to be used.

CONFUSION BETWEEN ART AND SCIENCE

John H. Musser (1850–1912), a good pathologist as well as clinician, carried the ideas of Cabot still further. In 1898, in a paper entitled "The Essential of the Art of Medicine," Musser, to a wearisome degree, stressed the importance of precision.[27] Older physicians did not use instruments of precision. Their diagnoses depended more on intuition and experience than on precise data. Musser condemned "intuition," which meant, "guessing the truth from ill-defined data," whereas accurate methods would make medicine inductive and rational.

For Musser, the proper method of inquiry involved "the application of scientific habits of thought in experiment, observation and analysis." This scientific habit of thought, together with instruments of precision, had "become essential in the practice of the art of medicine, in diagnosis and in therapeutics." Establishing a diagnosis might require a great deal of investigation, but "a close and severe method in gathering data," and orderly consideration of these data, coupled with use of instruments of precision, could make a diagnosis "scientific, precise and positive."

Therapeutics, to be scientific, must rest on experiment as the basis for conclusions. "To . . . conduct a judicious and productive therapeusis, two things are required, the scientific habit of mind and a scientific method of inquiry." Just as diagnosis required "patient, elaborate, precise inquiry," so too the same spirit must prevail in applying remedies.

So reasonable does all this sound that we may easily overlook the inconsistencies and fallacies. Musser had severe misconceptions regarding the nature of technology. He spoke of instruments "that deal only in truth," and in another place of "instruments of precision that cannot lie." Such blind faith in the validity of a "test" is, of course, the exact opposite of a "scientific habit of mind," and inconsistent with it. Musser used the word *art* with a pejorative reference, as virtually a synonym for *empiricism*. It referred to "chance methods" and vague experience and resulted from "intuition," which he condemned. He characterized the practice of the older physicians as art, meaning thereby that tools of precision were not available, or if available, were not used. On the other hand, when precise tools were used, Musser thought the art of medicine would be replaced by the science of medicine.

The notion that art could be replaced by science indicates a basic misconception. Musser ignored the age-old distinction, that science dealt with generalizations and universals, in the Platonic sense, while art concerned the treatment of the individual.[28] The art of medicine was involved when the physician pondered the question of which scientific principles would apply to a particular patient. In the science of medicine, the individual was no longer the central focus nor his or her welfare the sole consideration. Instead, the patient was a case, an instance, in some generalization. Art involved judgment and decision, which Hippocrates, almost 2,500 years before, had recognized as difficult. Since then, science has enormously multiplied the options, but the making of decisions and choices is still difficult.

Fortunately, the worship of laboratory precision aroused considerable criticism. In 1900, an editorial in the *Boston Medical and Surgical Journal* pointed out that the use of the word *scientific*, as applied to laboratory work, was establishing false standards.[29] Accuracy, to be sure, came largely through the laboratory. Yet the designation "scientific man" depended wholly on the attitude toward the problems whose solution required "the proper interpretation of those facts." The data may come from the laboratory, but "to study facts laboriously, and then appreciate clearly the meaning of those facts . . . and to make generalizations therefrom is, properly speaking, 'scientific.' " The editorial declared that "the present distinction between the scientific and practical physician was wholly false. . . . The 'scientific' physician is he who observes facts in a scientific manner." The author seemed to be saying that precision obtained in a laboratory was definitely an aid but by itself did not constitute science.

I call attention to another and correlative paper noting the pitfalls that could result from too much reliance on the laboratory. The author declared, "The first requisite for a diagnostician is not technical skill but a judicious mind, capable of weighing the value of evidence."[30] We readily see the difference between this viewpoint and Musser's naive faith in "instruments of precision that cannot lie."

RAPID ADVANCES IN CLINICAL SCIENCE

The development of clinical science in America, and its various European influences, are well described in A. McGehee Harvey's detailed account.[31] For this period, I will discuss only two episodes in the first decades of the new century.

First is the noteworthy lecture of Samuel J. Melzer (1851–1921) in 1909, presented when he became the first president of the American Society for Clinical Investigation.[32] The new society developed from the American Association of Physicians and became known colloquially as the "young Turks." Historians have raised questions whether there was a rebellion against the older physicians of waning enthusiasm. In Ellen Brainard's view, the new society arose because younger men were cultivating laboratory methods not familiar to the older elite.[33]

Draper, as we have seen, maintained that clinical medicine— "practical medicine"—if suitably investigated, could be as "scientific" as any medical science. A new breed of clinicians was studying the general principles of disease in the living patient while adhering to the canons of science. For Draper, the investigations did not require laboratory work, but in the twenty years following his paper a vast array of precise laboratory methods effected a transformation. New techniques were multiplying so rapidly that older physicians could not keep abreast. Younger men, skilled in using these tools, constituted the new society.

In clinical medicine, Melzer stressed the two distinct components, the science *and* the art. To some extent, he said, these are mutually antagonistic, and the simultaneous cultivation of both is detrimental to the progress of either. Science seeks "truthful knowledge," and any "motive of utility obscures its vision." Practice, on the other hand, uses the acquired knowledge "for the purpose of obtaining some useful end." Clinical science should be separated "from the mere practical interests."

Physicians who wanted to teach and to engage in academic medicine should, Melzer thought, have an education and training "radically different" from what prevailed earlier. For academic medicine, according to Melzer, clinical research and the extension of knowledge formed the major aspects. He made clear the inconsistencies between such a goal and the practice of medicine. He pointed to the research and educational activities in Germany as a model. We are reminded of the recommendations that Osler made in 1895 regarding the training that the modern academic clinicians should have.

CONFLICT BETWEEN THE OLD AND THE NEW

The career of David Linn Edsall (1869–1945) exemplifies the conflicts between the old and the new. Especially pertinent are the difficulties he faced in Philadelphia, when he was slated to succeed James Tyson as professor of medicine.[34] Edsall had studied chemistry in college and developed a strong interest in the basic sciences. He received his M.D. degree from the University of Pennsylvania in 1893. After an internship and a brief period of private practice in Pittsburgh, he returned to Philadelphia, where he could work in the new William Pepper Laboratory. He saw patients, engaged in research, and published extensively.

In seven years, Edsall wrote forty-two papers, in part clinical case reports but chiefly topics in clinical investigation, especially those that entailed chemical studies.[35] His contributions dealt with metabolic disorders, urinary constituents, gout, acromegaly, and diseases of the liver, among others. He was soon recognized as one of the outstanding younger men, a leader in the new type of clinical investigation.

He was slated to become head of medicine at the University of Pennsylvania, with a free hand to reorganize the departments. As a condition of acceptance, he insisted on the retirement of James

Tyson, whom we met earlier in this chapter. Tyson, the incumbent professor, was the leading physician in the city and beloved by patients, students, and faculty. Edsall's demand raised such a storm in Philadelphia that he withdrew from the appointment.

The episode illustrates well the changing views regarding the art and the science of medicine. This becomes clear if we glance at Tyson's record. He had received his M.D. degree from the University of Pennsylvania in 1863, and in the subsequent thirty years he became an outstanding clinician who embodied all the progressive tendencies of his generation. Although he had been well-trained in pathology, he regarded this subject not as an area for independent research but only as a stepping-stone to eminence in clinical medicine.

Among Tyson's many publications were a book on cell theory, published in 1870, entitled *The Cell Doctrine, Its History and Present State*, followed in 1873 by *Introduction to Practical Histology*. That same year he published *A Guide to the Practical Examination of the Urine*, which went through eight editions in twenty years, and expanded from 50 to 272 pages. Other publications include *Bright's Disease and Diabetes* (1881) and *A Manual of Physical Diagnosis*, (1891). These I have not consulted. His *Practice of Medicine*, mentioned earlier, bore the subtitle, *A text-book for practitioners and students with special reference to diagnosis and treatment*.

In 1876 Tyson was appointed professor of pathology and morbid anatomy and, in 1889, clinical professor of medicine. On the death of William Pepper, Jr., in 1899, he became the professor of medicine. He was a founding member of the AAP, in 1885.

Tyson represented the *art* of medicine. Admirably versed in the science of his day, he used all his scientific knowledge in the care of patients and in the teaching of students. He was skillful in applying the knowledge already available, but he did not take part in advancing knowledge. Edsall, on the other hand, was valiant in promoting new knowledge. Moreover, he was adept in the new techniques of chemistry, which were becoming increasingly significant in clinical investigation.

Tyson, I suggest, was never a medical scientist. His field, in the terminology of Draper, was "practical medicine," the domain of medical art. Edsall, on the contrary, exemplified "scientific medicine," but how much of the art he possessed is not now apparent.

The contrast between Tyson and Edsall illustrates the generation gap and the changes that took place therein. Tyson, outstanding in the 1880s, was born in 1841. Edsall, outstanding in 1910, was born in 1869. A medical leader of one generation, however eminent, could not maintain himself indefinitely at the top of his profession. New techniques developed and knowledge kept expanding. Perhaps most important of all, new values crept in, values influenced by events that might have had little obvious or direct relation to medicine. When a new bandwagon rolled into town, only the younger men had the agility to clamber aboard.

A change was taking place in academic medicine, as the laboratory and the canons of experimental study became increasingly important. Research, especially in the laboratory, symbolized the new academic physician. Melzer, in 1909, urged that physicians who devoted themselves to research should not also engage in practice, but he did not spell out the basic rationale or the fundamental difference between medical science and medical practice. A scientist wants to promote knowledge. Whether those interests concern hormonal balance, immunological reactions, or enzyme activity, the patient is primarily a source of data from which valid general principles may emerge. The individual patient is merely a point on a curve. Such is the science of medicine.

In contrast, for medical practice, the cure of the patient is the entire goal. The practitioner must use the knowledge—the general principles—that the scientist has discovered, but the skill with which the practitioner applies this knowledge to the individual patient belongs to the art of medicine.

Thus conflict exists between the scientist and the practitioner. Melzer, aware of this, urged caution in mixing the two aspects of medical activity. The emerging awareness of this conflict, with all its professional and social complications, showed that twentieth-century medicine was replacing that of the nineteenth century. Today, at the end of the twentieth century, we are aware of the problem, but we have not solved it. We can hope that the solutions will come from the medicine of the twenty-first century.

10

The Continuity of Problems

Benjamin Rush, who died in 1813, can represent eighteenth-century medicine and its characteristic thought modes. William Osler, who retired from the American scene in 1905, can stand for nineteenth-century medical thinking. In this interval of approximately a hundred years, medicine underwent massive but gradual transformation, some stages of which I have tried to trace in this book.

By 1908 different ways of thinking were clearly beginning to manifest themselves, and we can perceive a slow metamorphosis into what I would call twentieth-century medicine. And now, in the 1990s, we see new changes that presage still further transformation in attitudes and thought modes. These, we may confidently assert, will characterize the twenty-first century.

A continuity of problems bound the eighteenth to the nineteenth centuries. The same problems have persisted in the twentieth century and, in all probability, will link the twentieth to the twenty-first. I will deal briefly with only two such questions. First, What is disease? And second, How do you identify it?

DIAGNOSIS AS THE IDENTIFICATION OF PATTERNS

In simplest terms, a disease is an aggregate of phenomena that cohere in a sort of pattern, as if some inner connection bonded them together. In this sense, disease is truly a *syndrome*, a "running together" of particular features, like the several horses of a single chariot. If we draw on Latin roots instead of Greek, we can speak of a *concurrence*. The individual features, if considered in isolation, would be *symptoms*. When they cohere and interact and form a temporal pattern, we can speak of a *disease*. A particular pattern will acquire a name as a sort of handle that makes discourse easier and facilitates diagnosis.

A few striking examples come readily to mind. Earlier I described Louis's work on pneumonia. The pattern of chills, fever, pain in the chest, cough, and rusty sputum had an individuality that marked it off from other diseases. So too with the chills and intermittent febrile course of intermittent fever, or malaria; or the course and eruption of smallpox. The manifestations of a disease, that is, the symptoms, seemed to interlock and thereby to create an entity that could be identified, named, and further studied.

Ancient physicians recorded many such patterns. In the course of 2,500 years, new ones have been discovered, old ones have undergone change. What was once considered a unity might have become differentiated into two or more separable diseases; or several patterns, thought to be distinct, might have merged into a new unity.

Clinical patterns, when first defined, derived from the striking and clear-cut cases that called attention to themselves. Such early patterns were far from precise. The descriptions provided various criteria, whose application, clear in some cases, would be doubtful in others. All too often, the symptoms did not conform precisely to the original configuration. If a pattern when originally described had, say, six major components, and a given patient presented only five, did the patient have the disease or not?

We can use the disease typhus, already extensively discussed, as our model. In the eighteenth century Cullen provided criteria that could identify this disease. He enumerated its contagious property, the increased heat (i.e., fever in our present-day sense), a pulse that was weak and often rapid, urine that showed no changes, a clouding of mentation, and weakness and prostration. Of all these, some might be more prominent than others, and some might be absent. Thus, a patient might have a strong pulse, instead of a weak one. Or, the urine might be scanty and highly colored.

Could the physician then confidently diagnose typhus? The pattern, if drawn entirely from clinical findings, lacked precision. It could give only an approximate identification.

Over the next 150 years or so, increased precision made discrimination sharper. I would offer a rough analogy. In school a nearsighted pupil has difficulty in making out words on the blackboard. The child sees a pattern but cannot decide just what it indicates or includes: the youngster cannot discriminate between, say, "mammy" and "nanny" or between "train" and "brain." Let the child now get suitable eyeglasses and immediately the patterns become sharp and discrimination easy.

I suggest a parallel to diagnostic patterns. The child's recognitions improved when a new factor, the eyeglasses, were introduced as a tool of precision. For the clinician, discrimination and recognition can be improved if new technical advances can bring greater clarity. Such input may stem from various sources. One would comprise so-called tools of precision, the fruits of technology in its broad sense. During the early nineteenth century, for example, physicians who used auscultation and percussion to study pulmonary diseases greatly expanded information about tuberculosis and pneumonia. The vast amount of new data, coupled with new insights, led physicians to reorganize the earlier patterns of these diseases.

Even more important, perhaps, than new technological input was a broadened intellectual horizon, whereby information from other disciplines was combined with the original clinical observations. In the early nineteenth century, pathology furnished especially significant additions. When physicians performed autopsies in large numbers and studied the morbid anatomy of diseases, they amassed much new relevant data. The discipline of chemistry was not so far advanced as was that of pathology, and while chemistry did advance the knowledge of disease patterns, its contributions developed more slowly. Not until the twentieth century did chemistry reach its full stature and replace morbid anatomy as the leading component of progress.

Another source for data was an indefinite area that would eventually comprise epidemiology, public health, and medical sociology. Some physicians and concerned laymen were noting that social features, like poverty and overcrowding, might play a part in epidemics, and that industrial hazards and toxic substances had a role in many diseases.

To illustrate all these changes, we refer again to the alterations that the concept of typhus underwent. Cullen defined typhus in clinical terms, so that clinical observation alone provided criteria for recognition. Actually, he was not quite sure whether he was dealing with a single entity or a condition that eventually might subdivide, but this possibility did not trouble anyone until the early nineteenth century. Then French physicians began to study intensively the morbid anatomy of the disease. Important conceptual changes resulted.

In the condition the French called typhus, postmortem examinations provided a new distinguishing feature, namely, localized anatomical changes in the bowel. Obviously, a criterion furnished by postmortem examination was not directly helpful to a clinician studying a patient at the bedside, but the data had to be included in any overall pattern and could provide indirect assistance.

Much confusion ensued. The disease that the French called typhus generally showed a cluster of anatomical changes, but the disease that the British called typhus did not, for the most part. Were there two distinct diseases, each with its own set of criteria? Or was there only one, which could manifest itself in different ways? In any disease, some manifestations might be more essential and important than others. How to tell?

This particular impasse was resolved through the work of Gerhard. In a controlled study, he showed that what the British called typhus was a quite different disease, clinically and pathologically, from what the French described. Hence, what was called typhus and considered a single entity actually represented two diseases, each of which could be characterized by quite different patterns. One would continue to be called typhus, the other received a variety of names, of which typhoid fever became the most widely accepted.

Gerhard's views were not immediately adopted. For almost two decades many physicians refused to accept his evidence. Instead, they maintained that typhus and typhoid fever were merely variants of a single entity. The respective patterns were not yet so clear that the unique nature of each would stand out unequivocally. If in many cases, there was uncertainty regarding diagnosis and differentiation, we must conclude that the disease entity was not adequately defined.

CAUSAL FACTORS AS CONFERRING SPECIFICITY

At this point we can see a gradual shift in attitude. Originally, the disease called typhus had been defined on purely clinical terms. After pathology furnished additional data, the pattern began to show a separation into two. The differentiation, however, was incomplete and not convincing to all experts in the field. The presence of symptoms and of anatomical changes—matters of empirical observation—was not enough to establish cogency. More was needed, namely, an explanation based on cause.

Physicians had tried to establish specificity—that is, a unique character that would not be confused with any other disease—through empirical observation alone. They had not succeeded. There had to be a shift from a mere empirical *description* to a rational *explanation*. This could take place if causal factors could be identified. These would then form the bond that explained the concurrence of individual factors.

A symptom, whether a delirium, a high fever, or an ulcer of the bowel, is a empirical datum. The causal relation, however, is never directly observed. An assertion that one object is the cause of another is always an inference. The asserted relationship is a rational construct that explains (i.e., clarifies and renders intelligible) particular observations. When physicians attend to causes, they are shifting from an empirical viewpoint to one of rationalism.

Medical history provides a continuous dialectic between the rational and the empirical viewpoints, first one school prevailing, then the other. The eighteenth century has been called the age of rationalism, while the nosology and positivism of the early nineteenth century emphasized the empirical attitude. The example of typhus illustrates the limitations of observation alone. Without reference to causes there was no complete assurance, no cogency, regarding the nature of the disease.

John Armstrong tried to focus attention on causes. He, and later others, suggested that the nature of the cause could determine whether a disease was specific or nonspecific. A disease was specific if it resulted from one and only one agency. In reciprocal fashion, a cause would be specific if it induced one and only one disease.

The physicians of the time did not appreciate the full range of difficulties, for they failed to realize that specificity of cause was inseparable from specificity of effect. Causal factors would vary in their degree of specificity. Cold and dampness, for example, could have a role in many quite different diseases and, therefore, were entirely nonspecific. A cathartic, such as jalap, could produce a diarrhea but could not be considered fully specific, since diarrhea might result from many other causes. On the other hand, strychnine would be a specific cause, since it alone produced the highly characteristic type of convulsion that could not be induced by any other drug. When we search for causes, we see how significant was the pattern that allegedly resulted therefrom, and how essential was the need to delineate this clinical pattern as sharply as possible.

Serving as a model for specificity of disease was smallpox. Since the Middle Ages it had been recognized as having a unique character. The succession of symptoms, the nature of the eruption, the mode of spread, the phenomena of immunity, the considerable success in prevention (first by inoculation and later by vaccination) represented empirical observations. In the aggregate, they formed a complex pattern that seemed highly specific.

As explanation, physicians postulated some unique specific agent, called a contagion. This, we must realize, was not a matter of empirical observation but only a logical construct. It provided the bond that held together the elements of the pattern. The contagion was a postulated entity that alone induced smallpox, and smallpox could result from no other agent.

If smallpox had a specific agent as its cause, so too might other infectious diseases. However, one great difficulty intruded. When Armstrong wrote, the clinical findings of smallpox induced by the hypothesized agent were quite clear-cut, the pattern unusually distinct. With typhus this was not really the case, for its patterns were confused. A specific contagion might indeed be postulated as its cause; but if so, what were the supposed effects? There would have to be a well-defined total pattern, and this simply was not the case with typhus.

Over the next half century, extensive researches provided new relevant information from a variety of sources. After the original concept of typhus was recognized as a mixture of separable diseases, each of these was studied from various viewpoints—clinical, pathological, epidemiological, and immunological. As a result, different patterns emerged, each reasonably circumscribed. They justified physicians' hypothesizing specific agents (contagions).

The actual demonstration of such a postulated agent—the discovery, if you will—occurred only after the growth of bacteriology, as described in Chapter 7. Here was a relatively new discipline, which clarified the concepts of disease and opened the way for better explanations. There were, however, unexpected results.

The golden age of bacteriology, starting in the late 1870s, provided a fresh chapter in the study of disease. A possible causal agent might be not only postulated but actually demonstrated in empirical fashion and its properties examined. Typhoid fever offers a fine example of the complexities.

In 1880, in the lesions of this disease, histological study showed the presence of bacteria, described by Eberth (although previously seen by others). Four years later, these bacteria were successfully isolated and cultured. This alone did not determine whether they were causal, or concomitant, or an effect. A direct causal relationship had to be established. The so-called Koch's postulates, designed to prove causal efficacy, could not be fulfilled, for the disease could not be reproduced in animals. However, a high degree of correlation—with the bacteria present in virtually every case of the disease, and not found except in those cases—seemed enough to establish a causal relation.

By the end of the nineteenth century, assurance grew that the bacterium in question, long called Eberth's bacillus, played a causal role. Tests were developed for its identification, which could make the clinical diagnosis quite assured at a relatively early stage in the disease. The presence of the organism, together with the usual clinical findings, would assure the diagnosis. If the clinical findings were ambiguous, the presence of the bacillus removed all doubt.

However, in practice, the correlation between clinical manifestations and the presence of the bacterium was far from absolute. Some cases suggested typhoid fever clinically, but the bacillus of Eberth could not be identified. Instead, a comparable but clearly distinguishable bacillus might be found. There thus arose the concept of new disease pattern, called paratyphoid fever. It had many similarities to typhoid fever but was not identical with it. Two different types were discriminated, called paratyphoid A and paratyphoid B. They were identified not on clinical grounds but on bacteriological evidence.

During the first half of the twentieth century, the classification of enteric bacteria became highly complex. The relationships of genus, species, and varieties, which had vexed clinicians and nosologists, now troubled bacteriologists. The term *typhoid bacillus*, at one time considered adequate, no longer sufficed. The organism was then called a species of the genus *Eberthella*, then later a species of the much larger genus, *Salmonella*. The agents producing clinical paratyphoid fevers seemingly had a generic relationship to that of typhoid fever, as distinct species of this same genus.

The genus *Salmonella* had a huge number of species. Some were pathogenic to humans and could induce a great range of clinical findings. Some were primarily pathogenic for lower animals but might on occasion attack humans. The disease typhoid fever, while remaining distinct, became regarded as merely one specific type of the larger category called salmonellosis.

NEW METHODOLOGY FOR OLD PROBLEMS

At this point we must examine more closely the topic of etiology and its role in diagnosis. Typhus fever as described by Cullen had been discriminated into two distinct entities. This separation, which established typhoid fever as an entity, took place not through any reference to etiology but through the use of clinical, anatomical, and epidemiological features, alone.

Later in the century, physicians were able to discriminate between typhoid fever and paratyphoid fevers. This new identification represented important methodological advances over the earlier separation. The factor of cause now served as the differential feature that would distinguish two otherwise comparable patterns. Clinical findings alone were no longer adequate to discriminate the two diseases. Hence, the respective patterns, on which the diagnosis rested had to take account of the causal agent, not as a hypothetical entity but as an empirical datum that could be directly observed. The bacteria, the contagious principle, now provided the crucial differential feature.

Today, the bacterial (or viral) agent in infections is often called *the* cause of the disease. This, of course, is a logical error that older physicians scrupulously avoided. To speak of *the* cause of a disease, without qualification, ignores all other factors and commits the monocausational fallacy. Every event results from multiple causal factors of varied character. Hence, for meaningful discourse we must consider the kind of cause. Older physicians tried to identify these various kinds, or categories, through terms like *remote, predisposing, proximal, continuing, adjuvant,* and the like.

Within this traditional background, the bacteria in question do indeed have a special role: they provide truly rigorous discrimination. Their identification confers a specificity to the disease not otherwise obtainable. By analogy with other kinds of cause, as enumerated above, we can call the specific bacterium the *defining* cause of the disease. Through it we identify the disease as a discrete entity and can make an accurate differential diagnosis.

In any diagnostic pattern, some aspects are more important than others. We call any aspect defining or essential when diagnosis cannot be made without it.

By the late nineteenth century, experienced physicians could, with reasonable assurance, distinguish typhus from typhoid fever on clinical grounds alone. When doubt existed, demonstration of the microorganism would settle the matter.

In contrast, the distinction between typhoid and paratyphoid fevers could be made only by demonstrating the bacterium. The bacterium, part of the total disease pattern, thus has an *essential* quality that is mistakenly called *the* cause, without qualification. A more proper term would be the *defining cause.*

The discovery of bacteria and their causal relation to disease allowed scientists to make exquisitely fine discriminations and to find answers for many problems that had troubled earlier physicians. Nevertheless, certain basic problems persisted. Eighteenth-century observers, trying to discriminate one disease from another and to find rigorous differential features, used the terms *species* and *varieties.*

In early nosology, a disease species could not be subdivided. Its properties set it apart as a separate entity, not to be confused with any other. When, however, diseases seemed somewhat similar, with no means of making a sharp distinction, were they really separate, or was one a variety of the other? In some instances this problem might have only academic interest, but in others, important practical differences in treatment might result. Proper discrimination could profoundly affect therapy.

We no longer use the term *species* in reference to disease, but the implicit problem still remains. An example that has extended into recent times involved the relations between phthisis (representing pulmonary tuberculosis) and scrofula (tuberculosis primarily affecting the cervical lymph nodes). While the two conditions generally differed in their clinical pattern, sometimes the one seemed to pass into the other.

Was scrofula a separate disease or a variety of phthisis? Much excellent study in the nineteenth century tried in vain to find an answer. Koch's discovery of the specific tubercle bacillus seemed to settle the question, but only for a short time. Further work soon distinguished two distinct species. One, identified as *Mycobacterium tuberculosis*, had a predilection for humans, the other, *M. bovis*, for cattle. Scrofula resulted when the bovine species attacked humans, usually young children, through infected milk. The correct discrimination had important therapeutic and public health importance. Scrofula could by eliminated through appropriate public health measures that had no bearing on pulmonary tuberculosis.

There is still no objective measure to determine whether physicians are dealing with two diseases or with varieties of the same disease. We might, perhaps, say that the answer is of no importance, especially since we now have antibiotic therapy that is highly effective in both. This, however is a totally unhistorical attitude.

A second instructive example concerns pneumonia, at one time regarded as a single disease. There is no need to take up the rapid growth in our knowledge and in the way different patterns were discriminated. I refer only to what is ordinarily called lobar pneumonia induced by the pneumococcus, a disease much studied in the nineteenth century. In the twentieth century, one of the greatest scientific advances was the discrimination of the pneumococcus into numerous specific types, identified by complex serological means. Some types were far more prevalent than others, some more virulent than others. Significant for our purposes is the differing response to specific therapy.

Against some types of pneumococcus, appropriate techniques

could create specific antisera that served as quite effective therapy. The specificity, however, was marked. An antiserum that would act quickly on the appropriate type of pneumococcus would exert no effect on a different type. Moreover, for some types, effective antisera could not even be prepared. And as a still further complication, the number of recognizable types was constantly increasing, as new techniques developed.

Since effective specific therapy was available for certain types, the identification of that type was clearly important in therapy. Prompt administration of an appropriate effective antiserum might save the life of the patient.

The different types of pneumococcus would, perhaps, represent varieties of the same organism, and the resulting patterns would then be merely varieties of a single disease entity. But the relative patterns of behavior could be so different that the question troubling eighteenth-century nosologists was still intrusive. Did the different types identify different diseases? With lobar pneumonia, the question lost any practical importance when new therapy was discovered.

With my third example, however, the problem of the disease entity cannot be shunted aside. In the nineteenth century, the discovery of the gonococcus brought unity and precision into the disease pattern long known as gonorrhea. When penicillin proved so effective in therapy, it seemed as if the disease might be entirely eliminated—a vain hope, for after a while penicillin-resistant strains developed and blunted the original therapeutic promises.

Modern medicine has powerful new therapies, undreamed of in the eighteenth century. Today, the response to therapy is a major part of any disease pattern. When two conditions have many similarities, a difference in therapeutic response is taken into account. If we have two patients, each infected with gonorrhea, and one responds to antibiotics while the other does not, we may fairly ask the question. Do they both have the same disease?

We return to the problems that intrigued eighteenth-century doctors and led to formal nosology. The impetus was basically practical: How can we identify the disease from which the patient suffers? Physicians wanted to reach a diagnosis and to institute appropriate therapy. Diagnosis required first of all a series of classes, called diseases, each with its own identifying pattern. If the patient presented features that, in their essentials, matched the pattern defining the disease, the physician applied the name of that disease to the patient, thereby making a diagnosis.

Eighteenth-century nosologists drew up a complicated framework of definitions and relationships. While these earlier formulations no longer apply, the problems that called for such schemata are still fully operative. At great length, our modern textbooks discuss diseases, their causes, their definitions, their relations to each another, and the means of making discriminations. We constantly use the word *disease*—indeed, we cannot do without it. But what does it mean? This is not an otiose question.

The eighteenth century saw the first gropings into formal nosology. In the nineteenth century, such basic problems as classification, specificity, and causation became insistent and reached a substantial stage of development. They have formed a legacy for the twentieth century. Just as they have helped to shape our present thought modes, so will they continue to influence the new attitudes inevitable in the coming century.

There is a certain exhilaration in perceiving the successive stages of intellectual change and the factors that brought it about. We acquire a sense of continuity in history. We glimpse the different approaches to the same basic problems, and we appreciate the way technical advances laid the groundwork for new insights. We can see the truth implicit in the old French proverb, which I translate, the more things change, the more they remain the same.

Notes

1. A SURVEY OF RELEVANT PROBLEMS

1. Arthur W. E. O'Shaughnessy, "Ode," in *The Oxford Book of Victorian Verse*, ed. Arthur Quiller-Couch (Oxford: Clarendon, 1919), pp. 686–87.

2. Lester S. King, *The Medical World of the Eighteenth Century* (Chicago: University of Chicago Press, 1958).

3. See Thomas S. Kuhn, *The Structure of Scientific Revolutions* (Chicago: University of Chicago Press, 1962).

4. James Bryan, *Progress of Medicine During the First Half of the Nineteenth Century* (Philadelphia: Grattan and M'Lean, 1851). An "Introductory Lecture" that was "Published by the Class."

5. Lester S. King, *The Philosophy of Medicine: The Early Eighteenth Century* (Cambridge: Harvard University Press, 1978), pp. 64–93.

6. A good survey will be found in Frederick Lawrence Holmes, *Claude Bernard and Animal Chemistry: The Emergence of a Scientist* (Cambridge: Harvard University Press, 1974). See also Robert E. Kohler, *From Animal Chemistry to Biochemistry: The Making of a Biochemical Discipline* (Cambridge: University Press, 1982).

7. Elisha Bartlett, *An Introductory Lecture on the Objects and Nature of Medical Science* (Lexington, Ky.: N. L. and J. W. Fineall, 1841).

8. John Duffy, *The Healers: The Rise of the Medical Establishment* (New York: McGraw-Hill, 1976), pp. 98, 109.

9. John Harley Warner, *The Therapeutic Perspective: Medical Practice, Knowledge, and Identity in America, 1820–1885* (Cambridge: Harvard University Press, 1986), pp. 83–161.

10. Bartlett, *Introductory Lecture*, p. 4.

11. Elisha Bartlett, *An Essay on the Philosophy of Medical Knowledge* (Philadelphia: Lea and Blanchard, 1844).

12. Ibid., p. 225.

13. Austin Flint, *Medicine of the Future* (New York: D. Appleton, 1886). See also "Medicine in 1886," *JAMA* 7 (1886): 127–29.

14. Quoted in Flint, *Medicine of the Future,* p. 8.

15. King, *Medical World,* chap. 1.

16. Ernst Mayr, *The Growth of Biological Thought: Diversity, Evolution, and Inheritance* (Cambridge: Harvard University Press, 1982), p. 32.

17. King, *Philosophy of Medicine,* pp. 216–17.

18. For a fine survey of therapy, see *Therapeutic Perspective.*

19. King, *Medical World,* p. 188.

20. Robert J. Richards, *Darwin: The Emergence of Evolutionary Theories of Mind and Behavior Change* (Chicago: University of Chicago Press, 1987), pp. 11–12. In this connection, see also Charles Rosenberg, "Woods or Trees: Ideas and Actors in the History of Science," *Isis* 79 (1988): 565–70.

21. George Rosen, "Critical Levels in Historical Process," *J. Hist. Med.* 13 (1958): 179–89.

22. James H. Cassedy, *Demography in Early America: Beginnings of the Statistical Method, 1660–1800* (Cambridge: Harvard University Press, 1969); also, Cassedy, *Medicine and American Growth, 1800–1860* (Madison: University of Wisconsin Press, 1986), pp. 35–39.

23. There is a vast literature on Daniel Drake. For orientation and entrance into the literature, I suggest the recent symposium published in *JAMA* 254 (1985): 2111–28, especially the following papers: Henry D. Shapiro, "Daniel Drake and the Crisis in Early American Medicine," pp. 2113–16; Arthur G. King, "Drake, the Many-Sided Physician," pp. 2117–19; and Charles D. Aring, "Daniel Drake and Medical Education," pp. 2120–22.

For early medical education in Kentucky, see in addition Robert Peter, *The History of the Medical Department of Transylvania University* (Louisville, Ky.: John P. Morton, 1905, Filson Club publication no. 20); Lewis J. Moorman, "The Influence of Kentucky Medical Schools on Medicine in the Southwest," *Bull. Hist. Med.* 24 (1950): 176–86.

2. SOME BASIC CONCEPTS OF EIGHTEENTH-CENTURY MEDICINE

1. William Cullen, *First Lines of the Practice of Medicine, Including the Definitions of the Nosology,* ed. Peter Reid (Edinburgh: Bell et al., 1816). The text has been published in many editions, all showing the same numbering of paragraphs. References are to paragraph number. The preface, however, does not have a numbered format, and the references indicate pages in this edition.

2. Lester S. King, *The Medical World of the Eighteenth Century* (Chi-

cago: University of Chicago Press, 1958); King, *The Road to Medical Enlightenment, 1650–1695* (New York: American Elsevier, 1963); King, *The Philosophy of Medicine: The Early Eighteenth Century* (Cambridge: Harvard University Press, 1978); King, "Stahl and Hoffmann: A Study in Eighteenth Century Animism," *J. Hist. Med.* 19 (1864): 118–30.

3. Cullen, *First Lines*, p. 13.

4. Benjamin Rush, "On the Means of Acquiring Knowledge," in *Sixteen Introductory Lectures* (Philadelphia: Bradford and Inskeep, 1811), pp. 340–62; quotation on pp. 360–61.

5. Cullen, *First Lines*, p. 23.

6. Quoted in King, *Philosophy of Medicine*, pp. 251–52. This is my own translation from Boerhaave's Latin test, *Praelectiones Academicae*, 5 vols. (Turin: 1743), par. 19. The standard translation, *Dr. Boerhaave's Academical Lecture on the Theory of Physic*, 2d ed., 6 vols. (London: 1751–57), is incorrect and unsatisfactory. With Boerhaave, as with Cullen, the standard form of reference is by numbered paragraphs, uniform in the numerous editions.

7. Thomas Percival, "Essay 1, The Empiric; or Arguments against the Use of Theory and Reasoning in Physic. Essay II, The Dogmatic; or Arguments for the Use of Theory and Reasoning in Physic," in *Essays Medical and Experimental*, 2d ed. (London: J. Johnson, 1772), pp. 1–54.

8. Boerhaave, *Academical Lecture* (1751), par. 34.

9. For explication of the nonnaturals, see L. J. Rather, "The Six Things Non-Natural," *Clio Medica* 3 (1968): 333–47; Saul Jarcho, "Galen's Six Non-Naturals," *Bull. Hist. Med.* 44 (1970): 342–47; Jerome J. Bylebyl, "Galen on the Non-Natural Causes of Variation in the Pulse," *Bull. Hist. Med.* 45 (1971): 482–85; P. H. Niebyl, "The Non-Naturals," in ibid., pp. 486–92.

10. Cullen, *First Lines*, pp. 19, 20.

11. Lester S. King and Marjorie C. Meehan, "A History of the Autopsy," *Am. J. Path.* 73 (1973): 514–44.

12. Esmond R. Long, *A History of Pathology* (1928; reprint, New York: Dover, 1965); Long, *The History of American Pathology* (Springfield, Ill.: C. C. Thomas, 1962).

13. John Baptist Morgagni, *The Seats and Causes of Disease, Investigated by Anatomy: In Five Books, Containing a Great Variety of Dissections, with Remarks*, trans. Benjamin Alexander, 3 vols. (London: Millar and Cadell, 1769).

14. Ibid., vol. 1, pp. 643–74.

3. INFLAMMATION AND FEVER

1. William Cullen, *First Lines of the Practice of Medicine, Including the Definitions of the Nosology*, ed. Peter Reid (Edinburgh: Bell et al., 1816), par. 235.

2. Walter B. Cannon, *Bodily Changes in Pain, Hunger, Rage, and Fear,* 2d ed. (New York: D. Appleton, 1920).

3. Cullen, *First Lines,* par. 239.

4. William Cullen, *Physiology* (pt. 1 of *Institutions of Medicine*), 3d ed. (Edinburgh: Elliot, 1785), par. 159.

5. Cullen, *First Lines,* par. 239.

6. William Pultney Alison, *Outlines of Pathology* (Edinburgh: Blackwood, 1833), p. xi.

7. John Bostock, *Elementary System of Physiology,* 2 vols. (Boston: Wells and Lilly, 1828); Robley Dunglison, *Human Physiology,* 2 vols. (Philadelphia: Cary and Lea, 1832).

8. Cullen, *Physiology,* par. 281.

9. Bostock, *Elementary System,* vol. 2, p. 317; see also *Outlines of Pathology,* p. xiii.

10. A. Philip Wilson [Philip], *A Treatise of Febrile Diseases,* 4 vols. (Winchester, Eng.: Robbins et al., 1800–1804). Wilson officially changed his name to A. P. Wilson Philip. The first American edition of this book was published in 1816. I have not seen it and have used the original British edition.

11. Ibid., vol. 3, p. 23.

12. William Cullen, *Synopsis Nosological Methodicae,* 2d ed. (Edinburgh: Kincaid and Creech, 1772), p. 227. See also Cullen, *First Lines,* immediately preceding par. 6. This edition has all the definitions from the nosology preceding the discussion of particular diseases.

13. William F. Bynum, "Cullen and the Study of Fevers in Britain, 1760–1820," in *Theories of Fever from Antiquity to the Enlightenment, Medical History,* Supplement No. 1 (London: Wellcome Institute, 1981), pp. 135–37; Dale Smith, "Medical Science, Medical Practice, and the Emerging Concept of Typhus in Mid-Eighteenth Century Britain," in ibid., pp. 121–34; Smith, "The Rise and Fall of Typhomalarial Fever: I, Origins," *J. Hist. Med.* 37 (1982): 182–220.

14. Cullen, *First Lines,* par. 32.

15. Whitfield J. Bell, Jr., *John Morgan, Continental Doctor* (Philadelphia: University of Pennsylvania Press, 1965); George W. Corner, *Two Centuries of Medicine: A History of the School of Medicine, University of Pennsylvania* (Philadelphia: J. B. Lippincott, 1965); Martin Kaufman, *American Medical Education: The Formative Years, 1765–1910* (Westport: Greenwood, 1976).

16. Wyndham Miles, "Benjamin Rush, Chemist," *Chymia* 4 (1953): 37–77; James Whorton, "Chemistry," in *The Education of American Physicians: Historical Essays,* ed. Ronald L. Numbers (Berkeley and Los Angeles: University of California Press, 1980), pp. 72–94.

17. David Hawke, *Benjamin Rush, Revolutionary Gadfly* (Indianapolis: Bobbs-Merrill, 1971); Carl Binger, *Revolutionary Doctor: Benjamin Rush, 1746–1813* (New York: W. W. Norton, 1966); L. H. Butterfield, ed.,

Letters of Benjamin Rush, 2 vols. (Princeton: Princeton University Press for the American Philosophical Society, 1951); Richard H. Shryock, "Benjamin Rush from the Perspective of the Twentieth Century," in *Medicine in the United States: Historical Essays* (Baltimore: Johns Hopkins Press, 1966), pp. 233–51.

18. For comments on bloodletting, see Lester S. King, *The Medical World of the Eighteenth Century* (Chicago: University of Chicago Press, 1958), pp. 149–50.

19. For an overview of John Brown's doctrines, see King, *Medical World,* pp. 145–49; Guenter B. Risse, "The Brownian System of Medicine: Its Theoretical and Practical Implications," *Clio Medica* 5 (1970): 45–51; Risse, "The Quest for Certainty in Medicine: John Brown's System of Medicine in France," *Bull. Hist. Med.* 45 (1971): 1–12.

20. Benjamin Rush, "Outlines of the Phenomena of Fever," *Medical Inquiries and Observations,* 4 vols. (Philadelphia: Johnson et al., 1809), vol. 3, p. 7.

21. Lester S. King, "What Is Disease?" *Phil. Science* 21 (1954): 193–203; King, "What Is Disease?" in *Concepts of Health and Disease: Interdisciplinary Perspective,* ed. A. L. Caplan, H. T. Engelhardt, Jr., and J. J. McCartney (Reading: Addison-Wesley, 1981), pp. 107–18; Charles E. Rosenberg, "Diseases and Social Order in America," in *AIDS: The Burden of History,* ed. Elizabeth Fee and Daniel M. Fox (Berkeley and Los Angeles: University of California Press, 1988), pp. 12–32.

22. Rush, "Outlines," p. 36.

23. Benjamin Rush, "On the Necessary Connection Between Observation and Reasoning in Nature," in *Sixteen Introductory Lectures* (Philadelphia: Bradford and Inskeep, 1811), pp. 1–16.

24. Henry Clutterbuck, *An Inquiry into the Seat and Nature of Fever* (London: T. Bussey et al., 1807), p. viii; Clutterbuck, "An Essay on Pyrexia, or Symptomatic Fever," in *Dunglison's American Medical Library, Medical and Surgical Monographs* (Philadelphia: A. Waldie, 1838), pp. 403–50.

25. Clutterbuck, *Inquiry,* p. 74.

26. Erwin H. Ackerknecht, *Medicine at the Paris Hospital, 1794–1848* (Baltimore: Johns Hopkins Press, 1967).

27. For listings of Broussais's writings, see Bayle and Thillaye, eds., *Biographie médicale par ordre chronologiqu,* 2 vols. (Paris: Delahaye, 1955), vol. 2, pp. 875–82; C. C. Gillispie, *Dictionary of Scientific Biography,* 10 vols. (New York: Scribner's, 1970–74), vol. 2, pp. 507–9; the American editions that I used are F. J. V. Broussais, *A Treatise on Physiology Applied to Pathology,* trans. John Bell and R. LaRoche, 3d American ed. (Philadelphia: Carey and Lea, 1832); Broussais, *Principles of Physiological Medicine,* trans. Isaac Hars and R. C. Griffith (Philadelphia: Carey and Lea, 1832).

28. Broussais, *Principles of Physiological Medicine,* prop. 70. Although

the propositions are numbered in Roman numerals, I give them in Arabic numerals.

29. John Eberle, "Observations on the Pathology of Fever, with Strictures on the Physiological Doctrine of Broussais," *West. J. Med. and Phys. Sci.* 4 (1831): 9–23.

30. *Autobiography of Charles Caldwell, M. D.*, with preface, notes, and appendix by Hariot W. Warner and new introduction by Lloyd G. Stevenson (New York: Da Capo, 1968).

31. Charles Caldwell, *An Analysis of Fever* (Lexington, Ky.: T. T. Skilman, 1825).

32. Herbert S. Klickstein, "Charles Caldwell and the Controversy in America Over Liebig's 'Animal Chemistry,'" *Chymia* 4 (1953): 129–57.

33. Caldwell, *Analysis of Fever*, pp. 62–63, 66.

4. THE SEARCH FOR SPECIFICITY

1. William Cullen, *Synopsis Nosologicae Methodicae*, 2d ed. (Edinburgh: Kincaid and Creech, 1772), p. 253; my translation.

2. William Cullen, *First Lines, of the Practice of Medicine, Including the Definitions of the Nosology*, ed. Peter Reid (Edinburgh: Bell et al., 1816), par. 70.

3. John Armstrong, *Practical Illustrations of Typhus Fever, of the Common Continued Fever, and of Inflammatory Diseases*, notes by Nathaniel Potter, 1st American ed., from 3d British ed. (Philadelphia: James Webster, 1821); and 2d American ed., with corrections and appendix (1822).

4. For detailed discussion of Boerhaave, Sauvages, and the origins of nosology, see Lester S. King, *The Medical World of the Eighteenth Century* (Chicago: University of Chicago Press, 1958), chaps. 3 and 7.

5. Armstrong, *Practical Illustrations* (1821), pp. 14, 15. Miasmas were discussed only minimally.

6. The best summary occurs in George B. Wood, *A Treatise on the Practice of Medicine*, 2d ed., 2 vols. (Philadelphia: George Eliot, 1849); see vol. 1, pp. 139–46.

7. John Armstrong, *Lectures on the Morbid Anatomy, Nature, and Treatment of Acute and Chronic Diseases*, ed. Joseph Rix, 1st American ed., with account of the life and writings of Dr. Armstrong by John Bell, 2 vols. (Philadelphia: DeSilver, Thomas, 1837).

8. Ibid., vol. 2, p. 107. For typhomalaria, see Dale Smith, "The Rise and Fall of Typhomalarial Fever: I, Origins," and "II, Decline and Fall," *J. Hist. Med.* 37 (1982): 182–220, 287–321.

9. Armstrong, *Lectures*, vol. 2, p. 107.

10. Carleton B. Chapman, *Dartmouth Medical School: The First 175 Years* (Hanover: University Presses of New England, 1973); *Dictionary of National Biography* (New York: Scribner's, 1935–36), vol. 9, pp. 324–27.

11. *Am. J. Med. Sci.* 15 (1834): 270–71.

12. Nathan Smith, *A Practical Essay on Typhous Fever* (New York: Bliss and White, 1824), reprinted in *Medical Classics* 1 (1937): 781–819. References are to the pagination in *Medical Classics.*

13. Jacob Bigelow, "On Self-Limited Diseases" lecture delivered in 1835, published in *Nature in Disease* (Boston: Ticknor and Fields, 1854), pp. 1–58.

14. W. F. Bynum. "Hospital, Disease, and Community: The London Fever Hospital, 1801–1850," in *Healing and History: Essays for George Rosen,* ed. Charles Rosenberg (London: Dawson; New York: Science History Publications, 1979), pp. 97–115; John M. Eyler, *Victorian Social Medicine: The Ideas and Methods of William Farr* (Baltimore: Johns Hopkins University Press, 1979); Royston Lambert, *Sir John Simon, 1816–1904, and English Social Administration* (London: MacGibbon and Kee, 1963).

15. Thomas Southwood Smith, *A Treatise on Fever* (London: Longman's, 1830); 1st American ed. (Philadelphia: Carey, Lea, and Blanchard, 1830). References are to pagination in the London edition.

5. THE SEARCH PARTLY SUCCESSFUL: THE DISCRIMINATION
OF TYPHOID FEVER

1. David Hosack, *A System of Practical Nosology,* 2d ed. (New York: Van Winkle, 1821). For a discussion of nosology, generally, see Lester S. King, *Medical World of the Eighteenth Century* (Chicago: University of Chicago Press, 1958), pp. 194–226; and King, *Medical Thinking, A Historical Preface* (Princeton: Princeton University Press, 1982), pp. 16–69.

2. M. A. Petit and E. R. A. Serres, *Traité de la Fièvre Entéro-mésentérique* (Paris: Hacquart, 1813).

3. King, *Medical Thinking,* pp. 16–69.

4. Leonard Wilson, "Fevers and Science in Early Nineteenth Century Medicine," *J. Hist. Med.* 33 (1978): 386–407; Pierre-Fidèle Bretonneau, *Traité de la Dothinentérie et de la Spécificité de Pierre-Fidèle Bretonneau,* with preface and notes by Louis Dubreuil-Chambardel (Paris: Victor Brothers, 1922), pp. 44–46.

5. Bretonneau, *Traité de la Dothinentérie,* pp. 243–74.

6. P. C. A. Louis, *Recherches anatomiques, pathologiques, et thérapeutiques sur la maladie connue sous les noms de gastro-entérite, fièvre putride, adynamique, ataxique, typhoide, ets. etc. Comparée avec les maladies aigues les plus ordinaires,* 2 vols. (Paris: J. B. Ballière, 1829).

7. J. Barnes, "Review of Louis, *Recherches Anatomique . . . 1829," Am. J. Med. Sci.* 4 (1829): 403–42.

8. Petit and Serres, *Traité de la Fièvre,* pp. 166–76.

9. P. Ch. A. Louis, *Anatomical, Pathological and Therapeutic Researches upon the Disease Known Under the Name of Gastro-enteritis,*

Putrid, Adynamic, Ataxic, or Typhoid Fever, Compared with the Most Common Acute Diseases, 2 vols., trans. Henry I. Bowditch (Boston: Hilliard, Gray, 1836).

10. Wilson, "Fevers and Science"; Dale Smith, "Gerhard's Distinction Between Typhoid and Typhus and Its Reception in America, 1833–1860," *Bull. Hist. Med.* 54 (1980): 368–85; for a contemporary survey of the relations of typhus and typhoid, see Marshall Hall, *Principles of the Theory and Practice of Medicine: First American Edition, revised and much enlarged by Jacob Bigelow and Oliver Wendell Holmes* (Boston: Little, Brown, 1839).

11. W. W. Gerhard, "Report of Cases treated in the Medical Wards of the Pennsylvania Hospital, Part 1st, Typhus and Remittent Fevers," *Am. J. Med. Sci.* 15 (1835): 320–42.

12. W. W. Gerhard, "On the Typhus fever, which occurred at Philadelphia in the spring and summer of 1836; illustrated by Clinical Observations at the Philadelphia Hospital; showing the distinction between this form of disease and Dothinenteritis or the Typhoid Fever with ulceration of the follicles of the small intestine," *Am. J. Hist. Med. Sci.* 19 (1837): 289–322; Gerhard, "On the Typhus Fever which occurred at Philadelphia in the spring and summer of 1836, Part second," *Am. J. Med. Sci.* 20 (1837): 289–322.

13. Gerhard, "On the Typhus Fever . . . Part second," p. 306.

14. Hall, *Principles*, pp. 239–59.

15. Elisha Bartlett, *The History, Diagnosis, and Treatment of Fevers of the United States*, 2d ed. (Philadelphia: Lea and Blanchard, 1847).

16. D. F. C. "Review of *The History, Diagnosis and Treatment . . . 1847*, by Elisha Bartlett," *Am. J. Med. Sci.*, n.s., 16 (1848): 396–406.

17. Joseph M. Smith, "Report of the Committee on Practical Medicine," *Trans. Am. Med. Assn.* 1 (1848): 101–33. See also "Domestic Summary," in *Am. J. Med. Sci.*, n.s., 16 (1848): 512–26.

18. Smith, "Report of the Committee," p. 114.

19. Henry F. Campbell, "An Inquiry into the Nature of Typhoidal Fever. Being a Consideration of Their Theory and Pathology, *Trans. Am. Med. Assn.* 6 (1853): 421–76.

20. Austin Flint, *A Treatise on the Principles and Practice of Medicine*, 4th ed. (Philadelphia: Henry C. Lea, 1873).

21. Austin Flint, "Account of an Epidemic Fever which occurred at North Boston, Erie County, during the months of October and November, 1843," *Am. J. Med. Sci.*, n.s., 10 (1845): 21–35.

22. Austin Flint, *Case Reports of Continued Fever* (Buffalo: Geo. H. Derby, 1852).

23. Ibid., p. 242; see also Bartlett, *History, Diagnosis, and Treatment*, pp. 266–69.

24. Flint, *Case Reports*, p. 245.

6. CONGESTIVE FEVER AND THE CLINICAL ENTITY

1. David Hosack, *A System of Practical Nosology,* 2d ed. (New York: Van Winkle, 1821).

2. John Mason Good, *The Study of Medicine,* 2d ed., 5 vols. (London: Baldwin, Cradock, and Joy, 1825). I have used this British edition. Good's classification of diseases is included.

3. John Eberle, *A Treatise on the Practice of Medicine,* 2d ed., 2 vols. (Philadelphia: John Grigg, 1831). Eberle was discussed in chapter 3.

4. Governer Emerson, "Vital Statistics for the decennial period from 1830 to 1840," *Am. J. Med. Sci.,* n.s., 16 (1848): 13–33.

5. Thomas Stewardson, "Observations on Remittent Fever, founded upon Cases Observed in the Pennsylvania Hospital," *Am. J. Med. Sci.,* n.s., 1 (1841): 289–384; ibid., n.s., 2 (1842): 277–98.

6. Dale Smith, "The Rise and Fall of Typhomalarial Fever, I, Origins," *J. Hist. Med.,* 37 (1982): 182–220.

7. John A. Swett, "On the Pathology of Remittent Fever," *Am. J. Med. Sci.,* n.s., 9 (1845): 29–51.

8. John W. Monette, "An Essay on the Summer and Autumnal Remittent Fevers of Mississippi," *West. J. Med. and Surg.* 1 (1840): 87–130.

9. Eberle, *Treatise on the Practice,* vol. 1, p. 73. Different authors offered variations on this picture.

10. Charles Parry, "Congestive Fever, Its Character, Symptoms and Treatment, as met with in Central Indiana," *Am. J. Med. Sci.,* n.s., 6 (1843): 26–33.

11. R. G. Wharton, "On the Congestive Fever of Mississippi, with Cases," *Am. J. Med. Sci.,* n.s., 7 (1845): 339–48.

12. Isaac Parrish, "Strictures on the use of the term Congestive as applied to the low forms of Fever," *Am. J. Med. Sci.,* n.s., 9 (1845): 283–308.

13. Marshall Hall, *Principles of the Theory and Practice of Medicine: First American Edition, revised and much enlarged by Jacob Bigelow and Oliver Wendell Holmes* (Boston: Little, Brown, 1839), pp. 28–91.

14. William J. Tuck, "On the Congestive Fever as Observed at Memphis, Tenn.," *Am. J. Med. Sci.,* n.s., 10 (1845): 334–37.

15. Samuel Dickson, *Essays on Pathology and Therapeutics,* 2 vols. (New York: Samuel and William Wood, 1845), vol. 1, pp. 290–91.

16. Charles E. Lavender, "Thoughts and Observations on Congestive Fever," *Am. J. Med. Sci.,* n.s., 16 (1848): 43–58.

17. Samuel Harvey Dickson, *Elements of Medicine: A Compendious View of Pathology and Therapeutics* (Philadelphia: Blanchard and Lea, 1855), p. 248.

18. George B. Wood, *A Treatise on the Practice of Medicine,* 5th ed., 2 vols. (Philadelphia: J. B. Lippincott, 1858), vol. 1, p. 311.

19. Austin Flint, *A Treatise on the Principles and Practice of Medicine,* 4th ed. (Philadelphia: Henry C. Lea, 1873), pp. 930–31.

20. Saul Jarcho, "Laveran's Discovery in the Retrospect of a Century," *Bull. Hist. Med.* 58 (1984): 215–44; Dale C. Smith and Lorraine B. Sanford, "Laveran's Germ: The Reception and Use of a Medical Discovery," *Am. J. Trop. Med.* 34 (1985): 2–20.

21. William Osler, *The Principles and Practice of Medicine* (New York: Appleton, 1892), p. 153.

22. James Tyson, *The Practice of Medicine* (Philadelphia: Blakiston, 1896), p. 69.

23. Paul Beeson and Walsh McDermott, eds., *Textbook of Medicine,* 14th ed. (Philadelphia: Saunders, 1975), p. 477.

24. James B. Wyngarden and Lloyd H. Smith, eds., *Cecil: Textbook of Medicine,* 17th ed. (Philadelphia: Saunders, 1985).

25. P. E. C. Manson-Bahr and F. I. C. Apted, *Manson's Tropical Diseases,* 18th ed. (London: Ballière Tindall, 1982), pp. 50–51.

26. Brian Maegraith, *Adams & Maegraith: Clinical Tropical Diseases* (Oxford: Blackwell, 1984), p. 279.

27. Richard K. Root and Merle A. Sande, *Septic Shock* (New York: Churchill Livingstone, 1985), pp. 2–3.

28. Wood, *Treatise,* vol. 1, p. 364.

29. Elisha Bartlett, *The History, Diagnosis, and Treatment of Fevers of the United States,* 2d ed. (Philadelphia: Lea and Blanchard, 1847), p. 352.

7. GERM THEORY, CAUSATION, AND SPECIFICITY

1. For general histories of bacteriology, see William Bulloch, *The History of Bacteriology* (London: Oxford University Press, 1938); W. D. Foster, *A History of Medical Bacteriology and Immunology* (London: Heinemann, 1970); C. E. A. Winslow, *The Conquest of Epidemic Disease: A Chapter in the History of Ideas* (New York: Hafner, 1967; facsimile of 1943 ed.); Herbert A. Lechavalier and Morris Solotorovsky, *Three Centuries of Microbiology* (New York: McGraw-Hill, 1965); Paul De Kruif, *Microbe Hunters* (New York: Harcourt Brace, 1926; Pocket Books, 1965).

2. Owsei Temkin, "An Historical Analysis of the Concept of Infection," in *The Double Face of Janus, and Other Essays in the History of Medicine* (Baltimore: Johns Hopkins University Press, 1977), pp. 456–71.

3. Elizabeth Fee and Daniel M. Fox, eds., *AIDS: The Burden of History* (Berkeley and Los Angeles: University of California Press, 1988).

4. John Armstrong, *Practical Illustrations of Typhus Fever, of the Common Continued Fever, and of Inflammatory Diseases,* notes by Nathaniel Potter, 1st American ed., from 3d British ed. (Philadelphia: James Webster, 1821), p. 268.

5. William Cullen, *First Lines of the Practice of Medicine, Including the Definitions of the Nosology,* ed. Peter Reid (Edinburgh: Bell et al., 1816), par. 81.

6. John Eberle, *A Treatise on the Practice of Medicine,* 2d ed., 2 vols. (Philadelphia: John Grigg, 1831).

7. Marshall Hall, *Principles of the Theory and Practice of Medicine, First American Edition, revised and much enlarged by Jacob Bigelow and Oliver Wendell Holmes* (Boston: Little, Brown, 1839).

8. See also Charles J. B. Williams, *Principles of Medicine, Comprising General Pathology and Therapeutics, and a Brief General View of Etiology, Nosology, Semeiology, Diagnosis, and Prognosis,* additions and notes by Meredith Clymer (Philadelphia: Lea and Blanchard, 1844).

9. Bigelow and Holmes, in Hall, *Principles,* p. 75.

10. For historical aspects of fermentation, see especially the relevant chapters in Bulloch, *History of Bacteriology,* and Winslow, *Conquest of Epidemic Disease.*

11. Thomas Watson, *Lectures on the Principles and Practice of Physic,* 3d American ed. from the last London ed., rev. with additions by D. Francis Condie (Philadelphia: Lea and Blanchard, 1847).

12. In this connection, see Winslow, *Conquest of Epidemic Disease,* p. 294.

13. Bulloch, *History of Bacteriology,* pp. 17–40.

14. Jacob Henle, "On Miasmata and Contagia," trans. George Rosen, *Bull. Inst. Hist. Med.* 6 (1938): 907–83; ref. to pp. 942–45.

15. Rudolph Virchow was the leading figure in this research. See Erwin Ackerknecht, *Rudolph Virchow, Doctor, Statesman, Anthropologist* (Madison: University of Wisconsin Press, 1953); L. J. Rather, *Addison and the White Corpuscles: An Aspect of Nineteenth Century Biology* (Berkeley and Los Angeles: University of California Press, 1872).

16. Henle, "On Miasmata," pp. 947–50.

17. Henry Holland, *Medical Notes and Reflections,* 2d ed. (London: Orme, Brown, Greene, and Longmans, 1840). I have used this edition, but have compared it with the first British edition of 1839 and the American edition of 1857.

18. Henle, "On Miasmata," pp. 943–44.

19. Williams, *Principles of Medicine.*

20. Alfred Stillé, *Elements of General Pathology: A Practical Treatise on the Causes, Forms, Symptoms, and Results of Disease* (Philadelphia: Lindsay and Blakiston, 1848).

21. Eberle, *Treatise,* vol. 1. p. 426; Elisha Bartlett, *The History, Diagnosis, and Treatment of Fevers in the United States,* 2d ed. (Philadelphia: Lea and Blanchard, 1847), p. 83.

22. Oliver Wendell Holmes, "The Contagiousness of Puerperal Fever"

(1843: rev. 1855), in *Medical Essays, 1842–1882* (Boston: Houghton, Mifflin, 1891), pp. 103–72.

23. An excellent account of classification of bacteria in its early aspects, is found in Bullock, *History of Bacteriology,* chap. 8.

24. For details, see ibid. plus the other texts in n.1, above.

25. Winslow, *Conquest of Epidemic Disease,* p. 302.

26. Gert Brieger has discussed the reactions of American surgery to Listerism and offered valuable comments on American bacteriological thinking of the period in "American Surgery and the Germ Theory of Disease," *Bull. Hist. Med.* 40 (1966): 135–45.

27. E. P. Hurd, "On the Germ Theory of Disease," *Boston Med. and Surg. J.* 91 (1874): 97–110; Thomas E. Satterthwaite, "Bacteria: Their Nature and Relation to Disease," *Medical Record* 10 (1875): 833–36; ref. to pp. 849–55; Phyllis Allen Richmond, "American Attitudes Toward the Germ Theory of Disease (1800–1880)," *J. Hist. Med. and Allied Sci.* 9 (1954): 428–54; Allen Richmond, "Some Variant Theories in Opposition to the Germ Theory of Disease," ibid.: 290–303; and Phyllis Allen, "Etiological Theory in America Prior to the Civil War," *J. Hist. Med. and Allied Sci.* 2 (1947): 489–520. Allen Richmond gives useful references, but her writings are marred by presentism.

28. Lester S. King, *The Medical World of the Eighteenth Century* (Chicago: University of Chicago Press, 1958), chap. 3.

29. Substantial extracts of Koch's original papers have been reprinted in translation in Lechavalier and Solotorovsky, *Three Centuries of Microbiology;* for the work on anthrax, see pp. 69–79.

30. Lester S. King, *Medical Thinking: A Historical Preface* (Princeton: Princeton University Press, 1982), pp. 55–64.

31. Koch's first paper on tuberculosis is most readily available in Robert Koch, "Die Ätiologie und die Bekämpfung der Tuberkulose," as reprinted in *Klassifer der Medizin,* ed. Karl Sudhoff (Leipzig: Barth, 1912), pp. 10–38. Portions are translated in Lechavalier and Solotorovsky, *Three Centuries of Microbiology,* pp. 85–109.

32. William T. Belfield, *On the Relations of Micro-organisms to Disease* (Chicago: W. T. Keener, 1884).

33. H. Gradle, *Bacteria and the Germ Theory of Disease* (Chicago: W. T. Keener, 1883).

34. Antoine Magnin, *The Bacteria,* trans. George M. Sternberg (Boston: Little, Brown, 1880).

35. Gradle, *Bacteria and Germ Theory,* p. 174.

36. James T. Whittaker, "Address in Medicine: Some Points in Bacteriology," *JAMA* 6 (1886): 533–44.

37. Henry D. Didama, "The Address in Medicine," *JAMA* 4 (1885): 505–9. For more on Didama, see Lester S. King, "The AMA Gets a New

Code of Ethics," Medicine in the U.S.A.: Historical Vignettes no. 9, *JAMA* 249 (1883): 1338–42.

38. J. J. Byrne, ed., *History of the Boston City Hospital, 1905–1964* (Boston: Boston City Hospital, n.d.), p. 304.

39. For a brief discussion of diphtheria, see Foster, *History of Medical Bacteriology,* pp. 71–74; and Lechavalier and Sotolorovsky, *Three Centuries of Microbiology,* pp. 122–34. The important role played by the New York City Board of Health is well covered in John Duffy, *A History of Public Health in New York City, 1866–1966* (New York: Russell Sage, 1974), pp. 97, 154–57.

40. J. C. Culbertson, "Diphtheria, Its Specific Diagnosis," *JAMA* 21 (1893): 698–99.

41. "The Early Diagnosis of Diphtheria," editorial, *JAMA* 25 (1895): 118–19.

8. CHANGING ASPECTS OF SCIENTIFIC MEDICINE, 1800–1850

1. Stanley Joel Reiser, *Medicine and the Reign of Technology* (Cambridge: Cambridge University Press, 1978).

2. For a discussion of Bacon's role in the modern scientific method, see Lester S. King, *Medical Thinking: A Historical Preface* (Princeton: Princeton University Press, 1982), pp. 269–71.

3. A sound discussion of positivism is presented by A. Robert Caponegri, *A History of Western Philosophy: Philosophy from the Romantic Age to the Age of Positivism* (Notre Dame: University of Notre Dame Press, 1971).

4. For a full discussion, see Lester S. King, *The Philosophy of Medicine: The Early Eighteenth Century* (Cambridge: Harvard University Press, 1978), pp. 233–58.

5. Erwin H. Ackerknecht, *Medicine at the Paris Hospital, 1794-1848* (Baltimore: Johns Hopkins Press, 1967).

6. William Middleton, "Samuel Jackson," *Ann. Med. Hist.,* n.s., 7 (1935): 538–49.

7. Samuel Jackson, *The Principles of Medicine Founded on the Study and Function of the Animal Organism* (Philadelphia: Carey and Lea, 1832).

8. Samuel Jackson, *A Lecture on Medical Education, Introductory to the Course of the Institutes of Medicine* (Philadelphia: 1833).

9. Jackson, *The Principles of Medicine,* p. x.

10. Jackson, *Lecture on Medical Education,* p. 15.

11. For the relation to Platonism, see Lester S. King, "Plato's Concepts of Medicine," *J. Hist. Med. and Allied Sci.* 9 (1954): 38–48.

12. William Osler, "Influence of Louis on American Medicine," *Bull. Johns Hopkins Hosp.* 8 (1897): 161–67.

13. P. C. A. Louis, *Researches on Phthisis, Anatomical, Pathological,*

and Therapeutical, 2d ed., trans. Walter Hayle Walshe (London: Sydenham Society, 1844); an advertisement to 1st ed. read, "dated 1825, and constituting a Preface"; Louis, "Memoir on the Proper Method of Examining a Patient, and of Arriving at Facts of a General Nature," trans. Henry I. Bowditch, in *Dunglison's American Medical Library, Medical and Surgical Monographs* (Philadelphia: A. Waldie, 1838); P. Ch. A. Louis, *Researches on the Effects of Bloodletting,* trans. C. G. Putnam, with preface and appendix by James Jackson (Boston: Hilliard, Gray, 1836).

14. Louis, "Memoir," p. 150.

15. Louis, *Researches on Phthisis,* p. xxiv.

16. Louis, "Memoir," p. 157.

17. Louis, *Researches on Phthisis,* p. xxiv.

18. Louis, "Memoir," pp. 163–65.

19. Louis, *Researches on . . . Bloodletting,* p. 8.

20. Both Cassedy and Porter have discussed Louis's shortcomings in statistical method, and also the impact of the numerical method on American medicine. Warner has given a particularly valuable account of the opposition of many American physicians to Louis's method. See James H. Cassedy, *American Medicine and Statistical Thinking, 1800–1860* (Cambridge: Harvard University Press, 1984), esp. pp. 54–67; T. M. Porter, *The Rise of Statistical Thinking* (Princeton: Princeton University Press, 1986), esp. pp. 152–62; John Harley Warner, *The Therapeutic Perspective: Medical Practice, Knowledge, and Identity in America, 1820–1885* (Cambridge: Harvard University Press, 1986), esp. pp. 197–206.

21. Louis, *Researches on . . . Bloodletting,* p. vii.

22. For information on American students in France in this period, see William Osler, "Influence of Louis on American Medicine," *Bull. Johns Hopkins Hosp.* 8 (1897): 161–67; Oliver Wendell Holmes, "Some of My Early Teachers," in *Medical Essays, 1853–1882* (Boston: Houghton, Mifflin, 1891), pp. 420–40; James Jackson, *A Memoir of James Jackson, Jr., With Extracts from His Letter to His Father; and Medical Cases, Collected by Him* (Boston: 1835); Russell M. Jones, "American Doctors in Paris, 1820–1861," *Bull Hist. Med.* 25 (1970): 143–57; Margaret Warner, "Letters from a Young Physician: James Jackson, Jr., and His Two Medical Fathers," *Harvard Med. Alumni Bull.* 60 (1986): 40–45.

23. Louis, *Researches on . . . Bloodletting,* pp. xxvii–xxviii.

24. For a general discussion of homeopathy, see Lester S King, *The Medical World of the Eighteenth Century* (Chicago: University of Chicago Press, 1962), pp. 157–91; Martin Kaufman, *Homeopathy in America: The Rise and Fall of a Medical Heresy* (Baltimore: Johns Hopkins Press, 1971); Joseph H. Kett, *The Formation of the American Medical Profession: The Role of Institutions 1780–1860* (Westport: Greenwood, 1980), pp. 132–64.

25. For the founding of the AMA, see Lester S. King, "The Founding

of the American Medical Association," Medicine in the U.S.A., Medical Vignettes no. 4, *JAMA* 248 (1982): 1749–52.

26. Jacob Bigelow, "On Self-Limited Diseases," (1835) in *Nature in Disease* (Boston: Ticknor and Fields, 1854); Nathan Smith, *A Practical Essay on Typhous Fever* (New York: Bliss and White, 1824), reprinted in *Medical Classics* I (1937): 781–819. References are to the pagination in *Medical Classics*. Warner, *Therapeutic Perspective*, pp. 28–32.

27. Holmes, "Currents and Cross-Currents in Medical Science," in *Medical Essays*, pp. 173–208; quotation on p. 203.

28. Holmes, "Homeopathy and its Kindred Delusions," in *Medical Essays*, pp. 1–102.

29. This judgment was expressed in the *Dictionary of National Biography* in the biographical account of Sir John Forbes.

30. I have used Forbes's original journal publication, "Homeopathy, Allopathy, and 'Young Physic,'" *Brit. and Foreign Med. Rev.* 21 (1846): 225–65. The two Philadelphia reprints are listed in the *Catalogue of the Surgeon-General's Library*, but I have not seen them.

31. King, *Medical World*, p. 171.

32. Forbes, "Homeopathy," p. 243.

33. William Osler, "Elisha Bartlett, A Rhode Island Philosopher," in *An Alabama Student, and Other Biographical Essays* (New York: Oxford University Press, 1908), pp. 108–58.

34. Josiah Bartlett, *An Inquiry into the Degree of Certainty in Medicine, and into the Nature and Extent of its Power Over Disease* (Philadelphia: Lea and Blanchard, 1848).

35. Elisha Bartlett, *An Essay on the Philosophy of Medical Science* (Philadelphia: Lea and Blanchard, 1844). For comments on this book, see Osler, "Elisha Bartlett"; Erwin H. Ackerknecht, "Elisha Bartlett and the Philosophy of the Paris Clinical School," *Bull. Hist. Med.* 24 (1950): 43–60. For less favorable comment, see [John Forbes], "Book Review of *An Essay on the Philosophy of Medicine*," in *Brit. and Foreign Med. Rev.* 20 (1845): 140–47; and also Lester S. King, "Medical Philosophy, 1836–1844," in *Medicine, Science and Culture: Historical Essays in Honor of Owsei Temkin*, ed. Lloyd G. Stevenson and Robert P. Multhauf (Baltimore: Johns Hopkins Press, 1960), pp. 143–59.

36. Elisha Bartlett, *An Introductory Lecture on the Objects and Nature of Medical Science* (Lexington, Ky: N. L. and J. W. Finneal, 1841).

37. Cassedy, *American Medicine*, pp. 66–67.

38. Bartlett, *Introductory Lecture*, p. 13.

39. Bartlett, *Essay*, p. 67.

40. See King, *Medical Thinking*, pp. 247–66, for a discussion on the nature of fact.

41. Robley Dunglison, *An Introductory Lecture Delivered to the Class of Institutes of Medicine in Jefferson Medical College, November 4, 1847*

(Philadelphia: 1847), p. 22. See also [Forbes], "Book Review"; and the rather vapid review in *Am. J. Med. Sci.*, n.s., 20 (1845): 141–44.

42. Alfred Stillé, *Elements of General Pathology: A Practical Treatise on the Causes, Forms, Symptoms and Results of Disease* (Philadelphia: Lindsay and Blakiston, 1848), pp. 25–48.

43. Bartlett, *Essay,* pp. 218–19.

9. MEDICINE AS ART AND SCIENCE, 1850–1912

1. Robert V. Bruce, *The Launching of American Science, 1846–1876* (Ithaca: Cornell University Press, 1987).

2. For a lengthy discussion of the AMA, see Lester S. King, "The Founding of the American Medical Association," Medicine in the U.S.A., Medical Vignettes no. 4, *JAMA* 248 (1982): 1749–52.

3. *Proceedings of the National Medical Convention held in New York, May 1846, and in Philadelphia, May 1847* (Philadelphia: AMA, 1847), p. 85.

4. Lester S. King, "Medical Education: The Early Phases," Medicine in the U.S.A., Medical Vignettes no. 2, *JAMA* 246 (1982): 731–34; King, "Medical Education: The AMA Surveys the Problems," Medicine in the U.S.A., Medical Vignettes no. 6, *JAMA* 248 (1982): 3017–21; King, "The Painfully Slow Progress in Medical Education," Medicine in the U.S.A., Medical Vignettes no. 7, *JAMA* 249 (1983): 270–74.

5. For data on this organization, see King, "Painfully Slow Progress"; Steven J. Peitzman, "Forgotten Reformers: The American Academy of Medicine," *Bull Hist. Med.* 58 (1984): 516–28.

6. Lewis H. Steiner, *Annual Address Before the American Academy of Medicine at New York, September 16, 1879* (New York: American Academy of Medicine, 1879).

7. For an account of the origins of the AAP, see James Howard Means, *The Association of American Physicians: Its First Seventy-Five Years* (New York: McGraw-Hill, 1961). I differ with Means's evaluation of other contemporary events and their relevance to the founding of the AAP; see Lester S. King, "The AMA Gets a New Code of Ethics," Medicine in the U.S.A., Medical Vignettes no. 9, *JAMA* 249 (1983): 1338–42; King, "The Changing Scene," Medicine in the U.S.A., Medical Vignettes no. 10, *JAMA* 249 (1983): 1897–1900; see also William G. Rothstein, *American Physicians in the Nineteenth Century: From Sects to Science* (Baltimore: Johns Hopkins University Press, 1972), p. 213; Burton J. Blaustein, *The Culture of Professionalism: The Middle Class and the Development of Higher Education in America* (New York: Norton, 1976).

8. James H. Cassedy, "The Microscope in American Medical Science, 1840–1869," *Isis* 67 (1976): 76–97.

9. For Tyson's appointment, see J. H. Clark, "The Development of a Pathological Laboratory at Blockley," *Medical Life* 46 (1855): 237–52;

James Tyson's textbook was *The Practice of Medicine: A text-book for practioners and students, with special reference to diagnosis and treatment* (Philadelphia: P. Blakiston, 1896).

10. Simon Flexner and James H. Flexner, *William Henry Welch and the Golden Age of American Medicine* (New York: Dover, 1966; original ed., 1941), pp. 70–71.

11. George Dock, "Clinical Science in the Eighties and Nineties," *Am. J. Clin. Path.* 16 (1946): 677–80.

12. John S. Billings, "Medical Education: Extracts from Lectures delivered before the Johns Hopkins University, Baltimore, 1877–1878," partially reprinted in *Bull. Hist. Med.* 19 (1938): 311–69.

13. William H. Draper, "On the Relation of Scientific to Practical Medicine," *Trans. Am. Assn. Physicians* 3 (1888): 1–8.

14. Edward Morman, "Clinical Pathology in America, 1865–1915: Philadelphia as a Test Case," *Bull. Hist. Med.* 48 (1984): 198–214. This is an excellent study and provides a good survey of the literature.

15. C. Neubauer and J. Vogel, *A Guide to the Qualitative and Quantitative Analysis of the Urine: Designed Especially for the Use of Medical Men*, 4th ed., trans. W. O. Markham (London: New Sydenham Society, 1863).

16. Saul Jarcho, "Laveran's Discovery in the Retrospect of a Century," *Bull. Hist. Med.* 58 (1984): 215–24; Dale C. Smith and Lorraine B. Sanford, "Laveran's Germ: The Reception and Use of a Medical Discovery," *Am. J. Trop. Mcd. Hyg.* 34 (1985): 2–20.

17. A. McGehee Harvey, Gert H. Brieger, Susan L. Abrams, Victor A. McJusick, *A Model of Its Kind*. Vol. 1, *A Centennial History of Medicine at Johns Hopkins*. Vol. 2, *A Pictorial History of Medicine at Johns Hopkins* (Baltimore: Johns Hopkins University Press, 1989).

18. William Osler, "The Haematozoa of Malaria," *Brit. Med. J.* 1 (1887): 556–62.

19. Frederic A. Washburn, *The Massachusetts General Hospital, Its Development 1900–1935* (Boston: Houghton-Mifflin, 1939), pp. 106–7.

20. Editorial, "The William Pepper Laboratory of Clinical Medicine," *Boston Med. Surg. J.* 133 (1895): 603–4.

21. William H. Welch, "The Evolution of Modern Clinical Laboratories," *Johns Hopkins Hosp. Bull.* 7 (1896): 19–24.

22. Henry M. Hurd, "Laboratories and Hospital Work," *Bull. Am. Acad. Med.* 2 (1896): 483–95.

23. C. N. B. Camac, "Hospital and Ward Clinical Laboratories," *JAMA* 35 (1900): 219–27.

24. William Osler, "President's Address," *Trans. Am. Assn. Physicians* 10 (1895): xi–xv.

25. A. L. Loomis, "President's Annual Address," *Trans. Am. Assn. Physicians* 8 (1893): xvi–xx.

26. A. T. Cabot, "Science in Medicine," *Boston Med. and Surg. J.* 137 (1897): 481–84.

27. J. H. Musser, "The Essential of the Art of Medicine," *JAMA* 30 (1898): 1487–94.

28. See Lester S. King, "Plato's Concepts of Medicine," *J. Hist. Med. and Allied Sci.* 9 (1954): 38–48.

29. Editorial, "The Scientific Physician," *Boston Med. and Surg. J.* 142 (1900): 701–2.

30. T. C. Janeway, "Some Sources of Error in Laboratory Clinical Diagnosis," *Medical News* 78 (1901): 700–706.

31. A. McGehee Harvey, *Science at the Bedside, Clinical Research in American Medicine, 1905–1945* (Baltimore: Johns Hopkins University Press, 1981).

32. Samuel J. Melzer, "The Science of Clinical Medicine: What It Ought to Be and the Men to Uphold It," *JAMA* 53 (1909): 508–12, reprinted in *J. Clin. Investig.* 38 (1959): 1796–1803. I will not take up such major events of the early twentieth century as the establishment of the Rockefeller Institute and its hospital or the changing of the guard at Johns Hopkins when Osler left in 1905. For the development of such research institutions, see especially Harvey, *Science at the Bedside;* and George W. Corner, *A History of the Rockefeller Institute, 1901–1953* (New York: Rockefeller University Press, 1964).

33. Ellen R. Brainard, "History of the American Society for Clinical Investigation, 1909–1959," *J. Clin. Investig.* 38 (1959): 1784–95.

34. The information on Edsall is derived chiefly from Joseph C. Aub and Ruth K. Hapgood, *Pioneer in Modern Medicine: David Linn Edsall of Harvard* (Boston: Harvard Medical Alumni Association, 1970); and George W. Corner, *Two Centuries of Medicine: A History of the School of Medicine, University of Pennsylvania* (Philadelphia: J. B. Lippincott, 1965).

35. Aub and Hapgood, *Pioneer in Modern Medicine,* provide a list of Edsall's publications.

Index

Designed by Martha Farlow

Composed by World Composition Services, Inc., in Primer

Printed by The Maple Press Company, Inc., on 60-lb. Glatfelter Eggshell Offset
and bound in ICG Arrestox A with Lindenmeyr Elephant Hide endsheets

Library of Congress Cataloging-in-Publication data

King, Lester S. (Lester Snow), 1908–
    Transformations in American medicine : from Benjamin Rush to William Osler /
Lester S. King.
        p.   cm.
    Includes bibliographical references.
    Includes index.
    ISBN 0-8018-4057-0 (alk. paper)
    1. Medicine—History—18th century. 2. Medicine—United States—History—
20th century. 3. Rush, Benjamin, 1745–1813. 4. Osler, William, Sir, 1849–1919.
I. Title.
    [DNLM: 1. Rush, Benjamin, 1745–1813. 2. Osler, William, Sir, 1849–1919.
3. History of Medicine, 18th Cent.—United States. 4. History of Medicine, 19th
Cent.—United States. 5. Pathology—history—United States. WZ 70 AA1 K5t]
R151.K56 1991
610'.973'09034—dc20
DNLM/DLC
for Library of Congress   90–4662 CIP